PAUL EHRLICH'S RECEPTOR IMMUNOLOGY: THE MAGNIFICENT OBSESSION

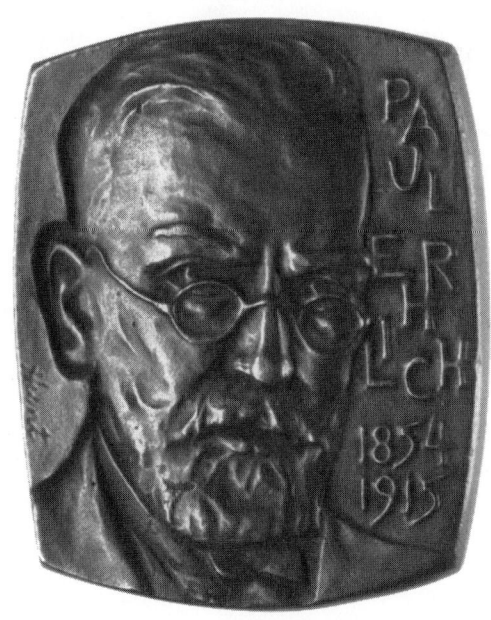

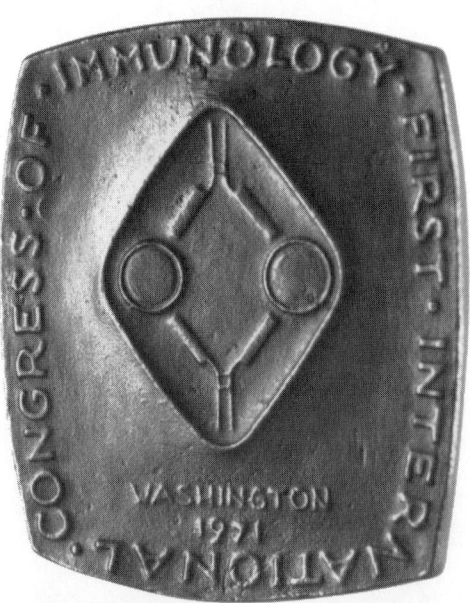

FRONTISPIECE   Medal honoring Paul Ehrlich, struck for the First International Congress of Immunology, Washington, D.C., 1971.

PAUL EHRLICH'S RECEPTOR IMMUNOLOGY: THE MAGNIFICENT OBSESSION

Arthur M. Silverstein

Institute of the History of Medicine
The Johns Hopkins University School of Medicine
Baltimore, Maryland

With an introduction by
Sir Gustav Nossal, *MD, PHD, FRS*

ACADEMIC PRESS

San Diego   London   Boston   New York   Sydney   Tokyo   Toronto

Academic Press
A Harcourt Science and Technology Company
525 B Street, Suite 1900, San Diego, California 92101-4495, USA
http://www.academicpress.com

Academic Press
Harcourt Place, 32 Jamestown Road, London, NW1 7BY, UK
http://www.academicpress.com

Library of Congress Card Number: 2001094613

International Standard Book Number: 0-12-643765-3

PRINTED IN THE UNITED STATES OF AMERICA
01 02 03 04 05 06 SB 9 8 7 6 5 4 3 2 1

To my wife Frances
and in memory of Günther K. Schwerin

CONTENTS

1

THE BACKGROUND TO EHRLICH'S IMMUNOLOGY: ORIGINS OF THE RECEPTOR THEORY

2

ON RICIN AND ABRIN: QUANTITATION ENTERS IMMUNITY RESEARCH

3

THE VALUE OF MOTHER'S MILK: THE FOUNDING OF PEDIATRIC IMMUNOLOGY

4

THE STANDARDIZATION OF TOXINS AND ANTITOXINS

5

THE TOXIN–ANTITOXIN REACTION: THEORY OUTPACES DATA 55

6

THE SIDE-CHAIN THEORY OF ANTIBODY FORMATION 77

7

IMMUNE HEMOLYSIS: BORDET CHALLENGES EHRLICH 95

8

NEW SCIENTIFIC CHALLENGES 123

9

EHRLICH'S SCIENTIFIC STYLE 137

List of Plates

INTRODUCTION

In this age of complex and wonderfully powerful technologies, it is easy to forget that scientific research is primarily about ideas. The fact that science is also about numbers, as Max Delbrück insisted, is somewhat less obvious. The best scientists build their experiments around an exciting hypothesis, using solid techniques and strict quantitation. A few carry a dominant infusing paradigm from one problem to others, fertilizing several research areas. A very few indeed reach the pinnacle again and again; for them we reserve the term genius and from them we must learn. A tiny handful achieve such luster as to outlive their era and shine on into history. One such, indubitably, is Paul Ehrlich. For this reason, a penetrating and sensitive analysis of his work is a major intellectual event. All serious observers of the triumphant scene that is modern immunology should therefore be very grateful to the distinguished immunologist and historian Dr. Arthur M. Silverstein for describing so clearly Paul Ehrlich's "magificent obsession."

Most immunologists would know Paul Ehrlich for three things: the introduction of quantitative methods into the study of antibodies and antigens; the side-chain theory, which was the distant forerunner of clonal selection; and the discovery of Salvarsan. Silverstein indeed summarizes and discusses these admirably, but he does much more. He places them into an unbroken chain of research, showing us wonderful work spanning a full 38 years. Furthermore, he reveals that a single preoccupation provided the thread linking quite disparate research endeavors, namely that biological processes depend on the interaction between a substance and a preformed receptor—an interaction that was specific and depended on stereochemical fit. Ehrlich remained faithful to this paradigm all his life.

We learn about Ehrlich's early work on staining reactions of tissues with dyestuffs, a chemistry-rich M.D. thesis in which the seeds of the idea of biological specificity are already apparent. This interest leads to the development of techniques to stain blood cells, with Ehrlich identifying basophils, eosinophils, and neutrophils. The basis is the staining of the granules of these polymorphonuclear leukocytes with basic, acidic (eosin being the typical one), or neutral dyes. The great Max Wintrobe therefore recognized Ehrlich as one of the fathers of modern hematology. Ehrlich also discovered how best to stain Koch's tubercle bacillus and briefly worked on tuberculin. Much more significant studies, however, were those on the plant toxins, ricin and abrin, in which Ehrlich first demonstrated his ability to introduce rigorous quantitation into immunity research—that is, the standardization of toxin activities and of antibody strength. These predated the work of Behring and Kitasato on the treatment of diphtheria by the passive injection of antitoxin antisera from various animals. It was logical and relatively simple for Ehrlich to apply the knowledge gained via the plant toxin system to the urgent questions of how to produce very high-titred sera and how to standardize the doses used in treatment. It was really Ehrlich's clinical trials that proved the value of Behring's discovery, which had previously been bedevilled by inconsistent and variable results. Furthermore, in the plant toxin studies, Ehrlich had essentially solved the problem of transfer of antibodies from mother to infant, showing that this involved both transplacental transport and passage of antibodies via the milk. Thus, he was in a position to use goat and cow milk as an alternative to serum as a source of antitoxin. This approach appears not to have been followed actively, and soon horse serum became the standard clinical tool, ruling the therapy of diphtheria for 30 years. Then, diphtheria toxoid was perfected and active immunization gradually took over.

The nature of the antigen–antibody interaction preoccupied Ehrlich greatly. Even famous men make mistakes. Thus, Ehrlich argued with Svante Arrhenius about the reversibility of the reaction, claiming that when antigen and antibody met, a chemical reaction akin to covalent bonding took place. Of course, in many situations that Ehrlich encountered, the bivalence (or multivalence) of antibodies made the reaction operationally irreversible. Ehrlich was also wrong in his argument with Jules Bordet about complement, claiming that immune hemolysis could not be explained without a multiplicity of complements. Dr. Silverstein produces a fascinating insight into Ehrlich's mind as he takes us through the elaborate contortions of theorizing, ad hoc argument piled on ad hoc argument, because of course Ehrlich thought that he was *always* right.

In no area was this self-confidence more apparent than in Ehrlich's side-chain theory. This held that antibodies were specific receptors on the cell surface, which preexist as natural molecules. When the antigen (e.g., a toxin) enters the body, it combines in a stereospecific manner with the receptor and neutralizes it, thus setting up a process whereby the body needs to make up for the deficiency by forming more receptors. With further injection of antigen, the process overshoots and excess natural antibodies spill into the serum. Silverstein sees the pictorial form of this theory, as presented in 1900 in Ehrlich's Croonian Lecture of the Royal Society, as epitomizing his magificent obsession and also as having been particularly influential. This side-chain theory was the crowning glory of Ehrlich's excursion into immunology. After 1901, his fertile mind and active laboratory research turned elsewhere.

Although Ehrlich's work on cancer, using various transplantable tumor models, was not particularly successful, his shift in 1905 into the chemotherapy of various infectious diseases provided the last glorious chapter of this remarkable scientific life. He used screening techniques and chemical modifications of promising compounds to attempt to find the "magic bullets" capable of killing pathogens while leaving the host unharmed. In June 1909, Ehrlich's faithful associate Sahashiro Hata, recently arrived from Japan, tested compound number 606 in a variety of infections. It soon proved capable of curing syphilis, and, with the drug christened Salvarsan, the modern era of scientific pharmacology was ushered in. Had he lived long enough, Ehrlich would surely have won a second Nobel Prize for this feat.

Silverstein concentrates on giving us a full and satisfying insight into Ehrlich's scientific *oeuvre*. He succeeds admirably in guiding us into looking at the various problems with the mindset of Ehrlich's times. He avoids going into details of Ehrlich's personal life except to the extent that Ehrlich the scientist is naturally influenced by Ehrlich the man. Chapter 9 is of particular interest as it explores Ehrlich's scientific style. Silverstein develops the theory that all Ehrlich's work rests on a single precept, namely the interaction of agonists with preformed receptors. But we learn much more than this. We gain insight into Ehrlich's temperament, his character, his leadership qualities, his interactions with scientific colleagues, indeed his *Weltanschauung*.

Those of us who have known Art Silverstein for many decades and have admired his contributions to his chosen branch of immunology wondered greatly about the increasing time he was spending since the late 1970s on the history of immunology. We saw a first vindication in his excellent 1989 work *A History of Immunology*. Now we have a further and most welcome dividend in the present extraordinary book, a work of scholarship, a labor of love, in fact an obsession in its own right. The book will enrich the wide readership it will surely receive. We can only hope that its certain success will stimulate further projects. Our past leaders still have so much to teach us!

G.J.V. Nossal
Melbourne
December, 2000

PREFACE

In 1989, I finished *A History of Immunology*.[1] It had taken 11 years of part-time activity stolen from my research laboratory obligations—obligations owed both to the Independent Order of Oddfellows who had endowed my Chair and to the National Institutes of Health who financed my research. The writing of the book proved so fascinating, and the book was so well received, that I felt that I must do another historical work in immunology. But 11 years was too long, and I no longer felt free to shortchange my laboratory research, so that I opted to retire from the laboratory to the Welch Medical Library, where Gert Brieger generously let me have a small office in the Johns Hopkins Institute for the History of Medicine.

Why should it have taken 11 years to write a general history of immunology, and especially one that did insufficient justice to such areas as allergy, complement, and natural immunity, and that stopped short of the startling developments that accompanied the immunobiological revolution of the late 1960s and 1970s? Much of the answer lay in the dearth of secondary literature in this field; up to that point, not many historians (or even immunologists) had written analyses of the events of the past that might have provided shortcuts to an understanding of the contributions of individuals, of the bases for scientific disputes, or of the reasons why some ideas succeeded and others failed. Thus, one had perforce to depend largely on the original literature and an one's own interpretations, hoping that one had covered the writings fully and interpreted correctly both their literal meaning and the between-the-lines implications.

Now, some 10 to 20 years later, the field of historical studies in immunology has attained a certain status among the subdisciplines of the history of the biomedical sciences. A critical mass of investigators now exists, including book authors Anne-Marie Moulin,[2] Alfred Tauber,[3] Pauline Mazumdar,[4] Tatyana

Ul'yankina,[5] and Leslie Brent;[6] collections edited by Deborah Jan Bibel,[7] Gilberto Corbellini,[8] Mazumdar,[9] and Richard Gallagher et al.;[10] and numerous papers by these authors as well as by Alberto Cambrosio and Peter Keating, Ilana Löwy, Craig Stillwell, and Nicholas Rasmussin. In addition, several journals now give occasional space to historical contributions,[11] or to the reminiscences of elder-statesmen immunologists.[12] History of Immunology workshops were held at the International Congresses of Immunology at Toronto, Berlin, and Budapest, where interested individuals exchanged views on important events in the history of immunology. Finally, the past few years have seen a number of international symposia on the subject.[13] Thus, one may safely conclude that the history of immunology has come of age.

During several years of research around the periphery of immunological history,[14] I cast around for a major project to occupy my time and interest. I remembered having described in my book the proximate stimulus for my entrance into the history of immunology[15]—the story of a manuscript I was given to review for *The Journal of Immunology* on the maternal transfer of antibody to the neonate by a 1970s author, who failed to mention that Paul Ehrlich had done the same study and obtained substantially the same results 80 years earlier. I went back to reread Ehrlich's papers[16] and found them truly remarkable! Not only had Ehrlich in 1892 solved the problem of maternal–fetal transfer of antibody *in utero* and of maternal–neonatal transfer via the milk—devising for the purpose some of the most elegant experiments of the 19th century[17]—but in one of the papers he had actually defined the kinetics of the primary and booster antibody responses. This work would not be improved on for a further 80 years.

Surely this work should have been more widely known, if not from the original reports then certainly from one of the many biographies of Paul Ehrlich. As I read through these biographies, it became apparent that neither in that of his adoring secretary,[18] nor in those of his admiring students or later celebrants of his fame[19] were the details of this extraordinary work to be found. Indeed, many of them did not even mention the pediatric studies at all. As I examined other of Ehrlich's immunological research, I found the same lack of attention in the biographies to the fine and important details of Ehrlich the scientist. Nowhere was it made clear why he had embarked on a given set of immunological studies, nor was attention drawn to their precision and elegance. There was little elaboration of the details of Ehrlich's results or of their exact significance both contemporaneously and during the long-term development of the field of immunology.

Only in two places does one find at least an attempt to explore the minutiae of Ehrlich's science. In Claude Dolman's treatment of Ehrlich in *The Dictionary of Scientific Biography,*[20] most of his important studies are mentioned, but not in great detail. Only in the Festschrift for Ehrlich's 60th birthday[21] did his more famous colleagues and students come close to detailing Ehrlich's experiments and their significance, and even many of these summaries are incomplete. But even incomplete, this Festschrift had never been translated from its original German, and thus is essentially unavailable to most modern scientists (and even to many modern historians). Indeed, many of Ehrlich's other important studies (e.g., the ricin/abrin work; the maternal–fetal/neonatal experiments) were not even deemed important enough to be included in the 1904 *Collected Studies in Immunity,*[22] or to have been translated in the three-volume collection of Ehrlich's works put together in 1957 by Dr. Fred Himmelweit of St. Mary's Medical School. London, under the supervision of Sir Henry Dale.[23]

Here was my project, clearly defined. I would attempt to provide the details and an interpretation of Ehrlich's immunological studies, segment by segment. For each of the immunological areas in which he worked, I would attempt, where possible, to indicate *why* he undertook the studies (i.e., the contemporary context), *how* he did the experiments (the experimental design), *what* results he obtained, and, as best I am able, *the significance* of his results, both contemporary and in the long term. Given the publication habits of 19th-century scientists, and especially the occasional turgidity of Ehrlich's scientific prose, I have taken certain liberties in recasting his results and adapting his data tables into a form more understandable, perhaps, to modern readers.

I decided, further, that I would deal only with Ehrlich the scientist, and leave Ehrlich the man to others. But it quickly became apparent that the "scientist" is frequently influenced by the "man." When we see Ehrlich jealous of his discoveries and fighting an Arrhenius or a Gruber against their attacks on his position,[24] or an Ehrlich so imbued by a sense of logic that he builds logically consistent but otherwise improbably complicated *ad hoc* structures to integrate new data into old theories (as he did to explain toxin–antitoxin neutralization curves[25] or the multiplicity of complements[26]), then aspects of the man emerge as well. To the extent that these traits are discernible in Ehrlich, they will be commented on in the last chapter on Ehrlich's scientific style.

To fully explain Paul Ehrlich's ideas, and especially why some of them have not survived the test of time, poses a curious historiographic challenge. Historians consider it a sin (called *presentism*) to bring modern knowledge to bear when discussing historical data and its interpretation. If an Ehrlich 'misinterpreted' some results because he could not have known *at the time* of the existence of some interfering substance or process, this should not be held to reflect on his intelligence or competence. However, the modern reader (and especially the expert in that field) deserves to be told what it was that actually produced the misleading results, so that the reader may fully understand the experimental system, the data it produced, and thus why the historical interpretation was so reasonable.

This situation arises several times in the discussions of Ehrlich's work, most particularly in his (and others') studies of "anti-antibodies" and "anti-complements." In each instance, I will attempt fairly to explain why Ehrlich interpreted his data in a certain way and why, knowing what he did, the interpretations appeared to be both reasonable and logical. I will then point out what Ehrlich could not have appreciated at the time: the presence of unrecognized reagents and interactions that skewed the results to provide a false trail to the truth. This approach will, I hope, avoid the danger of seeming to judge Ehrlich using modern knowledge, while serving well the needs of the modern reader.[27]

I owe a strong debt of gratitude to many individuals whose assistance helped to smooth an otherwise problem-strewn path. Foremost among these is Günther Schwerin, last surviving grandson of Paul Ehrlich, whose recent untimely death is much regretted by his many admirers. Schwerin's friendship and enthusiastic support were invaluable; he not only sent me directly much important material on Ehrlich, but he provided me with an entry to the large collection of Ehrlich papers that he had deposited at the Rockefeller University Archives Center at Tarrytown, New York. He also established a fund there to support research on his grandfather's papers, from which I received a grant to defray the travel expenses incurred on many visits to the Archives Center. I acknowledge also the encouragement of Mrs. Elizabeth Brody, great-granddaughter of Paul Ehrlich, who has also generously supported the translation of many of Ehrlich's papers and of the Festschrift published in 1914 in honor of Ehrlich's 60th birthday.

At the Rockefeller Archives Center, I appreciated greatly the help of Dr. Darwin Stapleton, director of this well-equipped and well-organized institution, and of Dr. Lee Hiltzik, its archivist. I must also express my appreciation to Dr. Elizabeth Fee and the staff of the History of Medicine Division at the National Library of Medicine in Bethesda, Maryland, for their help in consulting their rich resources. I have also received valuable help from several others interested in Paul Ehrlich, notably Professor Dr. Hans Schadewaldt of Düsseldorf, Professor A. Thomas Stoeckl of Freiburg, Dr. Bernhard Witkop of Bethesda, and Gräfin Suzanne von Goertz of Munich.

I learned much about the arcana of immunological history from extensive discussions with Anne-Marie Moulin, Alberto Cambrosio and Peter Keating, Alfred Tauber, Noel Rose, and many others. I learned about problems of biography from Thomas Söderqvist (although we have agreed that what follows is not a biography; neither is it a hagiography). In the area of historiographic practices, I owe much to Gert Brieger, Harry Marks, Daniel Todes, Owsei Temkin, and Edward Morman for many instructive discussions.

NOTES AND REFERENCES

1. Silverstein, A.M., *A History of Immunology,* New York, Academic Press, 1989.
2. Moulin, A.-M., *Le Dernier Langage de la Médicine: Histoire de l'Immunologie de Pasteur au SIDA,* Paris, Presse Universitaire, 1991.
3. Tauber, A.I., and Chernyak, L., *Metchnikoff and the Origins of Immunology,* New York, Oxford University Press, 1991; Tauber, A.I., *The Immune Self: Theory or Metaphor?,* Cambridge, Cambridge University Press, 1994; Tauber, A.I. and Podolsky, S.H., *The Generation of Diversity: Clonal Selection Theory and Rise of Molecular Biology,* Cambridge, Harvard University Press, 2000.
4. Mazumdar, P.M.H., *Species and Specificity: An Interpretation of the History of Immunology,* New York, Cambridge University Press, 1995.
5. Ul'yankina, T.I., *Zarozhdeniye Immunologii [The Origins of Immunology],* Moscow, Nauka, 1994.

6. Brent, L., *A History of Transplantation*, London, Academic Press, 1997.

7. Bibel, D.J., *Milestones in Immunology*, New York, Springer, 1984.

8. Corbellini, G., ed., *L'Evoluzione del Pensiero Immunologico*, Torino, Bollati Boringhieri, 1990.

9. Mazumdar, P.M.H., *Immunology 1930–1980*, Toronto, Wall & Thompson, 1989.

10. Gallagher, R.B., Gilder, J., Nossal, G.J.V., and Salvatore, G., eds., *Immunology: The Making of a Modern Science*, New York, Academic Press, 1995,

11. For example, *Cellular Immunology, Immunology Today*, and *Nature-Immunology*.

12. For example, *Annual Reviews of Immunology, Immunology Today*, and *Annual Reviews of Biochemistry*.

13. Thus, *L'Institut Pasteur: Contributions à son Histoire*, M. Morange, ed., Paris, La Découverte, 1991; *Immunology: Pasteur's Heritage*, P.-A. Cazenave and G.P. Talwar, eds., New Delhi, Wiley Eastern, 1991; "Immunology as a Historical Object," *J. Hist. Biol.* 27(3): 1994; *Singular Selves: Historical Issues and Contemporary Debates*, A.-M. Moulin and A. Cambrosio, eds., Paris, Elsevier, 2001; see also *Hist. Philos. Life Sci.* 22(1): 2000.

14. Thus, "Ocular Immunology: On the Birth of a New Discipline," *Cell. Immunol.* 136:504, 1991; "The Pasteur Institute and the Advent of Immunology: The Great Immunological Debates," in: P.-A. Cazenave and G.P. Talwar, eds., *Immunology: Pasteur's Heritage*, Wiley Eastern Ltd., New Delhi, 1991, pp. 11–20; "The Structure and Dynamics of Immunology, 1951–1972: A Prosopographical Study of International Meetings," *Cell. Immunol.* 158:1, 1994; and "The Heuristic Value of Experimental Systems: The Case of Immune Hemolysis," *J. Hist. Biol.* 27:437, 1994.

15. *A History of Immunology*, note 1, pp. xi–xii.

16. Ehrlich P., *Z. Hygiene* 12:183–203, 1892; Brieger L. and Ehrlich P., *Deutsch. med. Wochenschr.* 18:393, 1892; Brieger L. and Ehrlich P., *Z. Hyg.* 13:336, 1893; Ehrlich P. and Hübener W., *Z. Hyg.* 18:51, 1894.

17. These experiments are described in Silverstein, A.M., *Nature Immunol.* 1:93, 2000.

18. Marquardt, M., *Paul Ehrlich als Mensch und Arbeiter*, Stuttgart, Deutsche Verlags Anstalt, 1924 (English ed., *Paul Ehrlich*, London, William Heinemann, 1949).

19. Lazarus, A., "Paul Ehrlich," in M. Neuberger, ed., *Meister der Heilkunde I*, Vienna, Rikola, 1922, pp. 9–88; Loewe, H., "Paul Ehrlich. Schöpfer der Chemotherapie," in *Grosse Naturforscher VIII*, Stuttgart, Wissenschaftlicher Verlagsges., 1950; Venzmer, G., *Paul Ehrlich, Leben und Werken*, Stuttgart, Mundus, 1948; Satter, H., *Paul Ehrlich, Begründer der Chemotherapie*, 2nd ed., Munich, Oldenbourg, 1963; Greiling, W., *Paul Ehrlich. Leben und Werk*, Düsseldorf, Econ Verlag, 1964; Bäumler, E., *Paul Ehrlich: Scientist for Life*, New York, Holmes & Meier, 1984.

20. Dolman, C., "Paul Ehrlich," in *Dictionary Sci. Biog.* 4:295–303.

21. Apolant, H., ed., *Paul Ehrlich: Eine Darstellung seines wissenschaftlichen Wirkens*, Jena, Gustav Fischer, 1914. This will be referred to henceforth as the *Ehrlich Festschrift*.

22. Ehrlich, P., *Gesammelte Arbeiten zur Immunitätsforschung*, Berlin, Hirschwald, 1904; English trans. by C. Balduan, *Collected Studies in Immunity*, New York, Wiley & Sons, 1906.

23. Himmelweit, F., ed., *The Collected Papers of Paul Ehrlich*, 3 vols., London, Pergamon, 1957–1960. There was to have been a fourth volume, but an extensive search has failed to reveal why it was never published. See Silverstein, A.M., *Bull. Hist. Med.* 75 No. 3, 2001.

24. *A History of Immunology*, note 1, p. 103 ff.

25. *A History of Immunology*, note 1, p. 97.

26. *A History of Immunology*, note 1, pp. 103 and 196.

27. I find moral support for this position in Nick Jardine's discussion of the uses and abuses of anachronism in writing the history of science (*Hist. Sci.* 38:251, 2000). He points out that if the intent is to understand what the historical figure *meant*, then "vicious anachronism" is a no-no; if, however, the intent is to explain a modern outcome, then there is "legitimate use of anachronism in the service of explanation and critique of past activities and products of the sciences" (p. 266).

1

THE BACKGROUND TO
EHRLICH'S IMMUNOLOGY:
ORIGINS OF THE
RECEPTOR THEORY

*...the sidechain theory was laid down fixed and finished in
the Sauerstoffbedürfnis [1885], at a time when there was not yet
an immunology.*

Leonor Michaelis[1]

It is undoubtdly rare that the general concept underlying a major breakthrough
in the biological sciences should have arisen suddenly and fully formed, like
Athena from the forehead of Zeus. More often, it is the slow accretion of many
varied facts that leads to a formulation that is tested and retested, each time
slightly modified, until a mature system of thought is acknowledged and made
explicit. So it was, among others, with Darwin's theory of evolution and with Vir-
chow's cellular pathology; so also was it with Paul Ehrlich's side-chain receptor
theory of antibody formation.

Thus, the epigraph by Michaelis, written in 1914 for the celebration of
Ehrlich's 60th birthday,[2] was his attempt to show that Ehrlich's theory had
grown on an earlier rootstock. But only five years later, Michaelis would unearth
Ehrlich's long-lost thesis for his M.D. degree,[3] entitled *Contributions to the Theory and Practice of Histological Staining,*[4] written in 1878. The discussion of
the mechanism of staining by this 24 year old put back to an even earlier date the
germination of the theory that would guide him in all of his future scientific
endeavors. We shall return to these two major contributions in due course, but
only after discovering that the seeds of his chemically based receptor theory had
been planted even earlier than this. To repeat the caveat mentioned in the preface, we shall examine Ehrlich's early science in detail, to look for the foundations of the theoretical system that he would apply so productively to so many

fields, commenting only briefly in passing on a few pertinent incidents from his private life.

SCHOOLING

Ehrlich was born in 1854 to a well-to-do middle-class family in Strehlen, Silesia, in what was at the time the southeastern part of Germany, now a part of Poland. He was sent to high school in Breslau where he excelled in Latin, mathematics, and the sciences (especially chemistry and biology), but apparently did poorly in more literary courses such as German composition. His future love of chemistry is presaged by his answer when asked to explain the meaning of his final exam essay in composition on the obligatory subject of "Life—a Dream." The young student stammered in distress, and finally came out with, "you know … life is … a chemical incident … a normal oxidation … and the dream … the dream is … a fluorescence of the brain."[5] Many years later, Ehrlich would write, "I really believe myself that my talents lie in the field of chemistry; I can picture the chemical formulae in my mental vision."[6] This is really a quite remarkable and probably rare talent. To look at a chemical formula on paper and "see" it mentally as a three-dimensional structure must be analagous to the architect who can look at the plans and "see" the finished building, or to the musician who can look at a fully scored page and mentally "hear" the music written.

As Ehrlich maintained his interest in chemistry, so also did he continue his love of Latin throughout his life. He would frequently utter or write a Latin aphorism in the course of his normal pursuits, and he addressed his cousin Carl Weigert affectionately as *Carolus Magnus,* and wrote letters to his colleague and friend August von Wassermann with the greeting *Lieber Aquaticus.*

While he was a student, young Ehrlich had the opportunity to visit his cousin Carl Weigert in the pathology department of the medical school in Breslau. Weigert had been one of the first to introduce the use of the newly discovered aniline dyes into histology. It was Weigert, 9 years Ehrlich's senior, who showed him stained tissue preparations and pointed out that some cells stain well while others stain only poorly or not at all—a demonstration that would be remembered later, with important consequences.

After completing high school, Ehrlich entered university in Breslau in 1872, to study medicine. Here he came under the influence of anatomist Wilhelm von Waldeyer, who exposed Ehrlich further to histological methods for the differentiation of cell types. When, shortly thereafter, Waldeyer was appointed to a professorship at the "newly refounded"[7] University of Strasbourg, he took Ehrlich with him. In Germany, a university student could transfer from one institution to another at will, thus tailoring an education to individual interests. Before he was done, Ehrlich's university travels would take him to Breslau, Strasbourg, back to Breslau, to Freiburg, back to Breslau again, and finally to present his thesis and take his degree at Leipzig. In this way, a student could study with the cream of

German medicine and science in a chosen area. Ehrlich, on his travels, would come under the influence not only of Waldeyer and his cousin Weigert, but also of chemist Adolph von Baeyer, botanist Ferdinand Cohn, and pathologists Julius Cohnheim and Rudolph Haidenhain. In Cohnheim's institute, Ehrlich would meet the American pathologist William Welch, the future Danish immunologist Carl Salomonsen, and the obscure country physician Robert Koch, who had come to Breslau to demonstrate his anthrax studies.

Throughout his medical student days, Ehrlich experimented with the wealth of new dyes emerging from the growing German chemical industry. He would test each dye on a variety of tissues, and under a variety of conditions, so that his benchtop presented a spectrum of colorful solutions, and his fingers and occasionally his face were colorfully smudged. In 1877, in anticipation of his doctoral thesis, the 23-year-old medical student published his first scientific paper, "Contributions to the Knowledge of Aniline Staining and Their Use in Microscopic Technics."[8] In this paper, Ehrlich described the technical aspects of tissue staining, and the variable staining qualities of a variety of tissues and cells. Interestingly, he devoted much of the paper to the study of the distribution of plasma cells in different tissues, and especially in the components of the lymphoid system: tonsil, peyers patches, regional lymph nodes, and spleen. Of course, he could have had no inkling of the future importance of these cells for the discipline of immunology.[9]

Then, the year after publication of this preliminary paper, Ehrlich offered up his histochemical magnum opus on the theory and practice of histologic staining, as a dissertation for the M.D. degree.[10] Part I bore the title "The Chemical Concept of Staining," and Part II "The Aniline Dyes and their Chemical, Technological, and Histological Relationships." This was a truly remarkable body of work, especially for a 24-year-old undergraduate. Its opening sentence defined well the current state of affairs in histology: "While in the modern histological literature, directions on tinctorial method are already so numerous, and still increase from day to day, yet their theoretical basis has had only a very negligible consideration." This sentence and the entire thesis testify not only to the current absence of chemical science in histologic technology, but also to the self-confidence that would characterize Ehrlich throughout his career. He, an outsider, would dare to introduce rigorous scientific method into this hitherto purely empirical field. Testifying also to Ehrlich's single-minded dedication to work, even as a student, is the story of his time in Leipzig while waiting for his degree. As a transient without a laboratory, he is said to have set up an experimental staining bench on the billiard table of the inn in which he roomed in order to continue his experiments.[11]

In this lengthy and fact-filled thesis, Ehrlich laid the basis for an understanding of the relationship between the chemical structure of dyes and their differential staining abilities. He reviewed the characteristics of numerous dyestuffs and discussed the importance of their ionic state, their concentrations and solubilities, and the solvents in which they could be used. He even commented on the impurities present in some of them and on the difficulties that certain impurities posed.

Three important points emerge from this early example of Ehrlich's approach to biological research, an approach that would characterize his future work in the several disciplines to which he would make important contributions:

The first point is chemical; staining reactions are purely chemical in nature rather than physical. (Twenty-odd years later, Ehrlich would argue for the chemical interaction between antibody and antigen against Jules Bordet's and Karl Landsteiner's physical adsorption ideas.)[12]

The second point of the dissertation is also chemical; there is discernible in staining reactions a certain degree of specificity, in that certain dyes react preferentially with certain cells or structures. (This implied that the dye attaches to some sort of receptor, based on charge or other characteristics.)

Finally, the third point is chemical as well; to a great extent, structure appears to define function. (The nature of the groups attached to the aniline core of the dye define not only molecular charge, but solubility and strength of attachment.)

Here was the seed of a receptor theory that would take fuller form, first in Ehrlich's 1885 cell respiration studies, then in his 1897 side-chain theory of antibodies, and finally in his ultimate triumph, the design of such pharmacological agents as Salvarsan, the future magic bullets of chemotherapy. As Michaelis pointed out, one learned from this dissertation how "the idea of the chemical binding of foreign substances to the protoplasm developed on reflection about the nature of staining, and how from this idea later developed the side-chain theory."[13] This point is even more fully developed by Maria-Louise Eckmann in her impressive dissertation on the historical significance of Paul Ehrlich's thesis. As well as indicating the critical importance of the work for future developments in histochemistry and hematology, Eckmann points out that "This idea [the chemical binding of substances to cells] dominated Ehrlich's life. A straight path led from the doctoral work past the significant publication *The Oxygen Requirements of the Organism* to vital staining, and further to the side-chain theory, whose experimental basis shaped the work on toxins, antitoxins, and immunity."[14]

It is noteworthy also that in this thesis Ehrlich reported the discovery and naming of the mast cell,[15] which would lead him naturally to later important discoveries in hematology, including the eosinophile, neutrophile, and basophile.

Given the fundamental importance to histology of Ehrlich's thesis, it is quite surprising that it was never published or even widely referred to in the staining literature. Perhaps it was too far in advance of its times and too radical a departure from contemporary practice to have been accepted in its entirety. However, Ehrlich's ideas on the science of histologic staining would attain wide acceptance over the succeeding decades as, in study after study, he slowly demonstrated the validity of his ideas. But in the meantime, his doctoral dissertation lay unremarked in the archives of the University of Leipzig for over 40 years, until Michaelis thought to search it out and bring it to the attention of the scientific community.

BERLIN

The Charité

Already known for his histologic staining, Ehrlich received an invitation to become an assistant in Professor Friedrich Frerichs's second medical clinic at the prestigious Charité Hospital in Berlin. The Charité was a teaching hospital in which the new relationship between chemistry and medicine was well recognized, and where basic and clinical research was encouraged. This was nowhere more evident than in Frerichs's department. Once the young Ehrlich had demonstrated his talent, Frerichs, whose favorite maxim was "Caged birds do not sing," allowed him even more time for research than was permitted to other assistants. How lucky the budding investigator was, not only to have a supervisor who encouraged research, but one who also let his students fly. As another of Frerichs's prominent students, Bernhard Naunyn, later said of his director,

> He accepted each one from the very first day as a man who unquestionably could and would do everything the position required of him. So confident was he, unfortunately, of this that he never gave us any instructions as to how we should do anything; indeed, he scarcely said what he wanted done. ... It was just as much a matter of course that we should make scientific investigations and produce able pieces of work, as that we should perform our clinical duties to his satisfaction. What this work should be and how we did it was again entirely up to us, for he let us come and go and do whatever we wished, however we wished.[16]

Whereas Naunyn might have been voicing a modest complaint at the lack of supervision, this situation well suited the imaginative Ehrlich. He never seemed to lack for interesting *and important* research projects, or for the time to pursue them. In the ten years during which he worked at the Charité, not only did he help found the new discipline of hematology by his description of the various blood leukocytes and by his groundbreaking studies on the anemias, but he opened up a new field of exploration with his monograph on cell respiration, *The Oxygen Requirements of the Organism,* to which we shall return. All this basic research was performed in the context of continuing clinical activities; during the same period, he published reports on syphilitic heart infarcts, on the occurrence and metabolism of glycogen in diabetics, on acute splenic tumor, and on phosphorus and iodine poisoning. Meanwhile, he found time to apply his knowledge of staining to a variety of different histologic problems, and to introduce for the first time the use of fluorescein to study aqueous humor dynamics in the eye.[17] Of further clinical importance, Ehrlich's diazo reaction for the detection of various substances in the urine[18] found broad acceptance in the diagnosis of a variety of febrile diseases, and his demonstration of supravital staining of peripheral nerve endings with methylene blue[19] was widely employed by neuroanatomists.

The papers Ehrlich published on this wide range of subjects point up another remarkable aspect of his modus operandi. He seemed to be aware of the important literature in each of these disparate fields, and never failed to cite those studies on which his work depended and those that his results contradicted.

Thus, he seemed to read everything in the medical literature, both from at home and abroad. This is testified to by the famous later photograph of his office in Frankfurt (Plate 13), in which a visitor could hardly find a seat because the desk, chairs, and even floor were covered by great stacks of books, journals, and reprints. In addition, he would shower his associates with notes suggesting that they read one or another scientific paper, or that "we must prepare an answer to so-and-so's recent statement."

Along these same lines, it is interesting to contrast the management styles of Frerichs with that of the Ehrlich who would later become an institute director. Where Frerichs took on bright young people and "let them sing [or fly]," paying little heed to what they were up to in the laboratory, Ehrlich oversaw everything closely. No matter how many assistants and students were working on different problems, Ehrlich would shower them daily with little notes (his famous *Blöke*) with questions, advice, and requests to "see the animals" or to "discuss the results." We shall return to this matter of Ehrlich's scientific style in Chapter 9.

The Oxygen Requirement of the Organism

Of all of Ehrlich's contributions during the period of the 1880s, this monograph[20] must be considered his most important. He prepared it as his *Habilitationsschrift,* or inaugural dissertation required for appointment as a university lecturer. Ehrlich once again had made an innovative technological contribution to medical research; he introduced the use of redox dyes to study intracellular physiology.

Ehrlich had previously demonstrated the specificity of dye interactions with cells, as we saw. Now he used the color changes that accompany the oxidation–reduction reactions of dyes to assess the oxygen-fixing capacities of various tissue cells in the body. The assumption was as follows: those cells that possess a high affinity for oxygen will provide a reducing milieu within the cytoplasm, whereas those that bind oxygen only poorly will provide an oxidizing environment. If, therefore, an oxidized (e.g., highly colored) dye is injected, it will maintain its color in cells that bind oxygen poorly. Similary, it will lose its color when reduced in cells that bind oxygen avidly. Alternatively, injection of the colorless reduced form of the dye will reveal those cells that oxidize well, since the dye will there become highly colored.

Ehrlich ascribed the specific physiological functions of the cell to a chemically conceived *Leistungskern* [activity- or power-nucleus]. The term was not intended to relate to the anatomic nucleus of the cell, but rather to something akin to the aniline nucleus of a complicated dye, where *side-chains* account for modifications of specific function. Once again, we see Ehrlich dealing in terms of structurally based specificity, of affinity,[21] and of side-chains (such as amino, nitro, and halogen groups) that determine solubility, color, and specificity. Michaelis was indeed correct; here in this 1885 paper, almost fully formed, was the preview of Ehrlich's famous 1897 side-chain theory. In Ehrlich's words, in living protoplasm a [chemical] nucleus of special structure is responsible for the specific function peculiar to the cell, and that to this nucleus are attached, as side-chains, atoms and atom-complexes which are of merely subordinate importance for the specific function of the cell, but not for its vital activity in general.[22]

But the final discussion in this monograph heralded another of Ehrlich's later interests, immunity to infectious diseases. Already he had come under the influence of Louis Pasteur and Robert Koch's advances in bacteriology, leading him to discuss the implications of his findings for cellular immunity to pathogenic organisms. Most bacteria require ample oxygen for life, so that those cells that bind oxygen strongly should provide a hostile (e.g., immune) environment for such organisms. Indeed, Ehrlich suggested explicitly that this thesis was not unlike that proposed by Ilya Metchnikoff to explain cellular immunity against infection, except that Metchnikoff's proposal involved only the mobile phagocytes, whereas Ehrlich's referred to parenchymal cells in general.

Hematology

In his book *Hematology: The Blossoming of a Science,* Maxwell Wintrobe suggests that it may always be difficult to say who has had the greatest impact on a field of science. But he immediately goes on to note that "the simple investigation that Paul Ehrlich conducted as a medical student … had consequences far more important than he dreamed. A new era in the history of hematology was initiated."[23] Elsewhere in the book, Wintrobe named Ehrlich the "father" of modern hematology. (He proposed that Ehrlich shares this honor with William Hewson [1739–1744], discoverer of the lymphatic system and of the nature of blood coagulation,[24] and with Georges Hayem [1841–1935], who described and systematized a number of hematologic disorders.)[25] The validity of Ehrlich's claim to paternity appears to be borne out in *Blood Pure and Eloquent,* a compendium of historical chapters in the history of hematology by some of its leading modern practitioners.[26] Here, it is the rare chapter on one or another aspect of hematology that does not pay tribute to Ehrlich, and indeed he is more frequently cited in the name index than any other individual.

Prior to Ehrlich's work on the blood, little quantitative knowledge was available. The structure of the circulatory system and that of the lymphatic system were known, the red and white corpuscles had been identified, and preliminary observations had been made on anemias and leukemias. Then came Ehrlich's demonstration of techniques for the staining of blood cells, which not only led directly to the development of clinically useful quantitative blood counts, but also attracted many to the study of the blood.

Throughout the period of the 1880s, Ehrlich continued his studies on the staining reactions of blood cells. In testing numerous aniline dyes on blood smears, he was able to distinguish and name basophiles whose cytoplasmic granules, like those of mast cells, take up basic dyes, and eosinophiles, whose granules take up acidic dyes (of which eosin is the prototype). Here was evidence that the intracellular elements of different cells might differ chemically, resulting in a degree of specificity in their staining reactions.[27] This idea was elegantly verified by Ehrlich in his demonstration that polymorphonuclear leukocytes possess granules that, while not stainable with either basic or acidic dyes, can be stained by colored neutral salts resulting from the combination of acidic and basic dyes—thus the term neutrophiles. Once again, the leitmotif of Ehrlich's work—chemical specificity depending on molecular structure—had been verified with outstanding results, in this instance an important contribution to the founding of a new medical discipline, hematology. He was also the first to distinguish between lymphogenesis in the spleen and erythrocyte and myelogenesis in the bone marrow. He also claimed, correctly, that contrary to popular notions, the lymphocyte is not the progenitor of the other leukocytes. From these studies came Ehrlich's important monograph *Color-analytical Investigations on the Histologic and Clinical Aspects of the Blood.*[28]

Ehrlich is as well known in hematology for his technical innovations as for his original discoveries. In introducing new staining methods, he maintained close contact with such dye chemists as Artur von Weinberg and August Laubenheimer, and even helped to design new derivatives with special characteristics. He originated the heat-fixation of blood smears, which improved their staining characteristics, an innovation that reveals well Ehrlich's originality. To determine the best temperature for fixation, he set up a copper plate with one end heated by a bunsen burner, thus establishing a temperature gradient along its length. He then tested slides dried at different positions, establishing that the optimum temperature for fixation was at that position on the plate at which a small drop of water would sizzle and evaporate rapidly.

As an important adjunct to his blood cell studies, Ehrlich also engaged in groundbreaking studies of various forms of anemia and leukemia. These included both clinical and laboratory investigations, and resulted in a lengthy series of reports, culminating in the publication with A. Lazarus and F. Pinkus of the definitive book *The Anemias.*[29]

There was a curious by-product of Ehrlich's anemia studies that resulted in his becoming the only nonrickettsiologist after whom a tribe and a species of rickettsia are named.[30] It happened that Ehrlich had a Russian assistant named Mikhail Georgievich Kurloff in his laboratory at the Charité in 1888. He assigned Kurloff to study the long-term effects of splenectomy on the blood of guinea pigs. Kurloff observed that some of the leukocytes in the splenectomized animals contained cytoplasmic granules. It was assumed that these granules were constitutive (i.e., normally occurring), like those of basophiles and eosinophiles. On returning to St. Petersburg, Kurloff published these observations in the local journal *Vratch* [*Doctor*],[31] mentioning that the work had been done "in the laboratory of Prof. Ehrlich in Berlin." Only some 30 years later were many of the newly identified rickettsial diseases shown to be accompanied by inclusion bodies within the infected cells of the host. The "Kurloff bodies" in the monocytes of the guinea pig were rediscovered by a Russian rickettsiologist S.D. Moshkovsky in 1937.

Moshkovsky ascribed these inclusions to infection of the guinea pig by an agent that he chose to name *Ehrlichia kurlovi,* "in honor of Paul Ehrlich, since it was in his laboratory that the first representatives of this group were discovered, and because he contributed so much to the study of the morphology of the blood and of the agents of infectious diseases."[32] How coincidental that the revision of rickettsial nomenclature should have been made by a Russian who, probably uniquely among rickettsiologists, had read and remembered the obscure paper published in Russian a half-century earlier.

WITH ROBERT KOCH

Ehrlich's life appeared to be amply rewarding during the early 1880s. He was becoming widely known and respected for his researches in histology and for his hematological studies, crowned for the moment by his publication of the *Oxygen Requirement* monograph. When Robert Koch described his discovery of the tubercle bacillus,[33] Ehrlich went immediately into his laboratory to devise a better staining method to reveal this organism.[34] In 1884, he was granted the honorary title of professor by the medical faculty of the University of Berlin, and in 1887 he received the prestigious Tiedemann Prize of the Senckenberg Scientific Research Society in Frankfurt. He had married Hedwig Pinkus from his native Silesia in 1883, and they had two daughters, Stephanie in 1884 and Marianne in 1886.

In 1885, Ehrlich's benevolent chief Frerichs died and was succeeded by Carl Gerhardt. Gerhardt was not opposed to medical research, but thought that his assistants should spend more time in the clinic than in the laboratory. Although many of Ehrlich's biographers describe him as uninterested in clinical affairs, this was probably not true; he was a good clinician, and always sought the clinical implications of his basic research. Nevertheless, his heart was always in the research laboratory. Thus, Gerhardt's appointment was bound eventually to make Ehrlich unhappy and frustrated. He would say later of that period, "When in those days I felt so miserable with Gerhardt, I always went to my dye cabinet and said, 'These are my friends, who will never forsake me.'"[35]

It is ironic that Paul Ehrlich, who had shown how better to stain Koch's tubercle bacillus, should have used that same stain in 1888 to detect tubercle bacilli in his own sputum. As his illness began increasingly to interfere with his work, the Ehrlichs decided to seek a rest cure in warmer regions. They left Berlin in the autumn of 1888 for Italy, and one must assume that Ehrlich was not completely unhappy to find an excuse to leave Gerhardt's supervision. From Lake Garda, they visited Naples, and thence to Egypt, where they spent time in Alexandria and Cairo and visited Luxor and Thebes. It was perhaps Ehrlich's only foreign travel that was not connected with a meeting or congress and the only period that Ehrlich spent not preoccupied with thoughts of experiments and science. He returned from these travels completely cured and ready to rejoin the scientific fray.

There was no thought of returning to the unhappy position at the Charité under Gerhardt. With the financial support of his father-in-law Joseph Pinkus, owner of a linen-weaving factory in Silesia, Ehrlich found some rooms near his Berlin apartment and opened up his own private research laboratory, even hiring a diener named Fritz. There he was able to continue his earlier investigations of aniline dyes, and to extend his studies on the relationship between chemical structure and biological activity. Using mice, he studied the derivatives of cocaine, "insofar as is possible, to determine the ultimate relationship between chemical constitution, local damage, and anesthetic activity." He was able to comment once again about these molecules that, "As is evident, the side-chains embody the carrier of specific activity."[36] He seemed especially interested in the toxic properties of cocaine, and developed his own method of administering the drug by feeding animals with biscuits soaked with solutions of the drugs and then dried, a technique that he would soon put to good use in his studies of plant toxins.

In the autumn of 1890, Robert Koch offered Ehrlich a position to supervise Koch's clinical tuberculosis unit at Berlin's Moabit municipal hospital, where Koch, the lion of Berlin medicine, had been given 150 beds for the treatment and study of tuberculosis. Not only was Koch already famous for his discovery of the life cycle of the anthrax organism and of the tubercle bacillus, but everyone expected his tuberculin to be the new cure of this dread disease. Koch was already negociating with the government for the construction of a new Institute of Infectious Diseases in Berlin, and when he moved into it in the summer of 1891, he took Paul Ehrlich with him. It is curious, however, that although Koch was very well supported financially by the government, Ehrlich was to work for him for more than three years without salary.

Tuberculin Studies

When Ehrlich went to work for Koch at the Moabit Hospital in 1890, he had already commenced his experiments on plant toxins several months earlier, in his private laboratory. Despite a busy clinical schedule with tubercular patients at the Moabit, he seems to have found time to continue these studies and bring them to a successful conclusion, as we shall see in the next chapter. For the moment, however, Ehrlich's principal obligation was to the treatment of tuberculosis.

Robert Koch had isolated from the fluid medium in which tubercle bacilli are cultured a substance that he named tuberculin. He had high hopes that this material, which he considered the toxic component of the tubercle bacillus, might serve as the cure of tuberculosis just as diphtheria and tetanus toxins were being shown by Behring and Kitasato to mediate the cure of these diseases. But while the early results with tuberculin therapy appeared promising, much more clinical experimentation was required by the cautious Koch to demonstrate conclusively its curative powers. Indeed, it was in part for this further testing that the large unit at the Moabit had been given to Koch.

Then, in one of the more unfortunate incidents in the history of medical research, the politicians in the Ministry of Culture and at the Kaiser's court strongly urged Koch to announce his "cure" to the world, at the upcoming International Congress of Medicine to be held in Berlin. This, it was felt, would once again demonstrate German leadership in medical research, strongly challenged by the recent successes of Louis Pasteur in France. Only at the end of a very general speech on bacteriological research did Koch make the startling announcement that after testing many chemicals, he had "at last hit upon a substance which has the power of preventing the growth of tubercle bacilli."[37] It is understandable that the announcement was received with great excitement; the end of the plague of tuberculosis was widely forecast. It would be all the more disappointing, then, when the coming years would show that not only did tuberculin treatment not cure the disease, but indeed it might cause occasional dangerous flare-ups of quiescent tubercles.[38]

Meanwhile, however, Ehrlich and other admirers of Koch attempted to define the parameters of usefulness of tuberculin. Almost all the reports start with a tribute to Koch's great discovery. The first study on the subject in which Ehrlich was involved was published in the *Berlin klinische Wochenschrift,*[39] one of many that would appear during the following several years. Ehrlich was junior author on this and several earlier preliminary reports, the senior being Paul Guttmann, director of the Moabit Hospital.

Guttmann and Ehrlich claimed that the fever response that was seen to follow the use of high doses of tuberculin is not critical to its therapeutic effect; therefore lower doses averting fever may be the best approach. This they demonstrate, giving slowly increasing doses of tuberculin every second day and noting an increase in weight in 32 of 36 patients, clearing of the lungs in some, and an overall improvement in most. (It must be appreciated that this was the period of euphoria about tuberculin therapy. Almost all publications initially reported a greater or lesser degree of therapeutic success with the *Koch'schen Heilungsmittel.*) Later, as reports of complications and less-than-satisfactory improvements in the condition of tubercular patients appeared, fewer and fewer physicians utilized tuberculin therapy, and indeed in some places the practice was prohibited.

It is probable that the use of initially low doses of tuberculin, with steady increase in dosage over time, was not an accidental observation. By the time tuberculin therapy was initiated at the Moabit, Ehrlich had already invented the method of small and steadily increasing doses of ricin and abrin to induce immunity in his private laboratory studies. He had found, as we shall see in the next chapter, that highly necrotizing lesions that accompany large doses of these toxins are not only undesirable, but unnecessary. Small doses are well tolerated, and induce in the test animals an increasing resistance to ever-larger challenge doses. If this works for these plant toxins, why should it not work for the putative toxin associated with the tubercle bacillus?

Ehrlich then summarized his work with tuberculin, and indeed his entire therapeutic philosophy, in a paper presented at the 1891 International Congress of Hygiene in London.[40] It was also a spirited defense of his much-admired chief, Robert Koch. In this manifesto on therapy, Ehrlich not only recommends his small-dose approach to tuberculin therapy, as published with Guttmann, but also outlines the guidelines that will govern all his future work in immunology, oncology, and pharmacology. There is, he states, a direct relationship between chemical structure and function; the binding of molecules by receptors mediates most of the functions of physiology. As Ehrlich says in the opening lines of the paper,

> Therapy, the most important branch of medicine, has from the outset developed on empirical grounds, in which more accidental or incidental observations on cures, be it in man or animal, led to the approach to practical use. Thus it was that the greatest majority of therapeutic substances have been attained, such as quinine, opium, and mercury. Only in recent times, especially with the progress in pure chemistry, have changes been made in this. One strives for the time when insight into the *essence* of drugs is attained, and to decide the question in the first instance of the relationship between the constitution of these substances and their *therapeutic* action. Justifying this approach was especially the more accurate research of the alkaloids, which showed that the great number of these variously active substances [have] a common nucleus similar to pyridine, to which side-groups connect as the carriers of physiological activity. This knowledge must necessarily lead to the desired goal of the synthesis of new drugs ... it will in fact be possible by means of certain combinations to eliminate nearby damaging activity without prejudicing the curative potency.

Here is the clearest statement thus far of the dream that Ehrlich would realize only some two decades later in his landmark excursion into scientific pharmacology.

The stage was now set for the imaginative Paul Ehrlich, steeped in structural chemistry, partial to quantitative methods, and with the seeds of a comprehensive theory of biological interactions already at hand, to tackle the problem of the mechanisms of immunity to toxins. He was, after all, generally interested in the pathogenesis of disease, and had previously studied the toxic effects of such substances as iodine, phosphorus, and cocaine. Perhaps it would be possible for Ehrlich to introduce quantitative chemical science into research on immunity, as he had introduced these methods in the fields of histology, hematology, and cellular physiology.

NOTES AND REFERENCES

1. Ehrlich, P., *Das Sauerstoffbedürfnis des Organismus, Eine Farbenanalytische Studie,* Berlin, Hirschwald, 1885. Reprinted in *Collected Papers of Paul Ehrlich,* Oxford, Pergamon, 1956, vol. I, pp. 364–432; English translation. pp. 433–496. These volumes will henceforth be referred to as *Collected Papers.*
2. Michaelis, L., in *Paul Ehrlich: Eine Darstellung seines wissenschaftlichen Wirkens,* Jena, Gustav Fischer, 1914, p. 25. This volume will hereafter be referred to as the *Ehrlich Festschrift.*
3. Michaelis, L., *Naturwissenschaften* 7:165, 1919.
4. Ehrlich, P., *Beiträge zur Theorie und Praxis der histologische Färbung.* Thesis, University of Leipzig, 17 June, 1878; *Collected Papers,* vol. I, pp. 29–64; English translation pp. 65–98.
5. Quoted in Marquardt, M., *Paul Ehrlich,* London, William Heinemann, 1949, pp. 11–12.
6. From Ehrlich's autobiographical notes, included in a letter to his friend Christian Herter, quoted in Marquardt, note 5, p. 15.
7. The Franco-Prussian War had just seen the defeat of France, with the reversion to German hands of Alsace, with its famous University at Strasbourg. (Louis Pasteur had been a professor there years before.) The enforced resignation of French professors opened up many faculty positions for German academics.

8. Ehrlich, P., *Arch. mikroscop. Anat.* 13:263, 1877; *Collected Papers,* vol. I, pp. 19–28.

9. It was finally Astrid Fagraeus who demonstrated that the mysterious plasma cell was in fact the source of circulating antibodies (*Acta Med. Scand. Suppl. No. 204,* 1948), a fact elegantly confirmed with flourescent antibodies by A.H. Coons, E.H. Leduc, and J.M. Connally (*J. Exp. Med.* 102:49, 1955).

10. See note 4. Ehrlich apparently chose Leipzig for his thesis defense because Cohnheim and Weigert, with whom he done much of his staining research, had recently moved to that university from Breslau.

11. Mentioned in W. Greiling, *Paul Ehrlich: Leben und Werk,* Düsseldorf, Econ-Verlag, 1954, p. 69. As Greiling says, "A gas connection and a water line—he did not need more. Rubber tubing, bunsen burner, glass vessels and chemicals he brought with him in his overcoat pocket."

12. For a description of these debates, see Silverstein, A.M., *A History of Immunology,* New York, Academic Press, 1989, p. 99 ff.

13. Michaelis, note 3, p. 168.

14. Eckmann, M.-L., *Die Doktorarbeit Paul Ehrlichs und ihre Bedeutung für die Geschichte der histologischen Färbung,* Dissertation, University of Hamburg, 1959, p. 26.

15. Ehrlich believed that these cells play a role in nutrition and chose the name from an old High German word *mästen,* to feed or fatten. It is related to the English word *meat.*

16. Naunyn, B., *Errinerungen, Gedanken, und Meinungen,* Munich, F. Bergmann, 1925, pp. 132 and 134; (English translation, *Memories, Thoughts, and Convictions,* Canton, Mass., Science History Publications, 1994). These comments quoted also by O. Temkin in the celebratory symposium on the 100th anniversary of Ehrlich's birth, *Bull. N.Y. Acad. Med.* 30:958, 1954.

17. Ehrlich, P., *Deutsch. med. Wochenschr.* 8:21, 35, 54, 1882; *Collected Papers* vol. I, pp. 344–353.

18. Ehrlich, P., *Z. klin. Med.* 5:285, 1882; *Collected Papers,* vol. I, pp. 619–629.

19. Ehrlich, P., *Deutsch. med. Wochenschr.* 12:49, 1886; *Collected Papers,* vol. I, pp. 500–508.

20. See note 1.

21. Ehrlich has apparently taken his concept of the *affinity* of oxygen binding to the cell from Pflüger's treatise, "Über die physiologische Verbrennung in den lebendigen Organismen," *Pflügers Arch. ges. Physiol. Mensch. Tier.* 10:251, 1875.

22. Ehrlich, *Collected Papers,* vol. I., p. 436.

23. Wintrobe, M., *Hematology: The Blossoming of a Science,* Philadelphia, Lea & Febiger, 1985, p. 25

24. LeFanu, W., "William Hewson," *Dict. Sci. Biog.* 6:367, 1972.

25. Verso, M.L., *Med. Hist.* 5:239, 1961.

26. Wintrobe, M., ed., *Blood Pure and Eloquent,* New York, McGraw-Hill, 1980.

27. Ehrlich, P., *Arch. Anat. Physiol. (Physiol. Abt.),* pp. 571–579, 1879; *Collected Papers* vol. 1, pp. 117–123.

28. Ehrlich, P., *Farbenanalytische Untersuchungen zur Histologie und Klinik des Blutes,* Berlin, Hirschwald, 1891. This is a collection of 13 of the publications on blood by Ehrlich and some of his collaborators and students.

29. P. Ehrlich and A. Lazarus, *Die Anämie,* Vienna, Hölder: Part I., Normale und pathologische Histologie des Blutes, 1898; Part II, Klinik der Anämien, 1900; Part III, (with F. Pinkus), Leukämie, Pseudoleukämie, und Hämoglobinämie, 1901; Part I was published in English translation in *Collected papers,* vol. I, pp. 181–268.

30. I was stimulated to search out this story by reading in the *New York Times* an article about an outbreak of the disease "Ehrlichiosis," an unfamiliar name whose possible relationship to Paul Ehrlich intrigued me. The story is presented in greater detail in Silverstein, A.M., *Bull. Hist. Med.* 72:731, 1998.

31. Kurloff, M.G. (in Russian), *Vratch [Doctor]* 10:515, 538, 1889.

32. Moshkovsky, Ch., *C. R. Soc. Biol.* 126:379, 1937. Nine years later, Moshkovsky published a new classification of rickettsiae (Moshkovsky, Sh. D. *Uspekhi Sovremennoi (Moscow)* 19:1, 1945 [in Russian]) that included not only the genus *Ehrlichia* but a family *Ehrlichiaceae,* since revised to a tribe *Ehrlichieae* (Philip, C.B., *Can. J. Microbiol.* 2:261, 1956; see also *Bergey's Manual of Systematic Bacteriology,* 9th ed., 1984, vol. I, p. 704).

33. Koch, R., *Berlin klin. Wochenschr.* 19:221, 1882. An English translation with a forward by A.K. Krause appeared in *Amer. Rev. Tuberculosis,* 25:285, 1932.

34. Ehrlich, P., *Deutsch. med. Wochenschr.* 8:269, 1882; *Collected Papers* vol. I, pp. 311–313.

35. See note 6; quoted by Marquardt, p. 28.

36. Ehrlich, P., *Deutsch. med. Wochenschr.* 16:717, 1890; *Collected Papers* vol. I, pp. 559–566. It is of interest that this paper was identified only as "by Prof. Dr. Paul Ehrlich in Berlin." The private laboratory was not deemed important enough to be included in the list of addresses of those papers originating from "Clinics, Hospitals, and Medical and Scientific Institutes." However, the ricin and abrin studies, though also done in his private laboratory, were listed as originating from the Institute of Infectious Diseases, to which Ehrlich had moved just prior to publication.

37. Koch, R., Tenth International Congress of Medicine, Berlin, August, 1890; reported in *Deutsch. med. Wochenschr.* 16:756, 1890; English translation in *Brit. Med. J.* 2:380, 1890. Koch followed up this announcement with further reports: *Deutsch. med. Wochenschr.* 16:1029, 1890; 17:101, 1189, 1891.

38. Koch believed that the toxic effects of tuberculin would act on the tubercles to effect their necrosis and thus kill the bacilli involved therein. However, these "focal reactions" in the eye and elsewhere often proved more harmful than the disease itself. This story is well discussed in Arnold Rich's *The Pathogenesis of Tuberculosis,"* 2nd ed., Springfield, IL, Charles C. Thomas 1944, p. 555 ff.

39. Guttmann P. and Ehrlich, P., *Deutsch. med. Wochenschr.* 17:793, 1891; *Collected Papers,* vol. II, pp. 7–12. 1891. See also Guttmann and Ehrlich, *Deutsch. med. Wochenschr.* 17:737, 1891.

40. Ehrlich, P., *Proceedings VII International Congress of Hygiene and Demography,* London, 2:211, 1891; *Collected Papers* vol. I, pp. 13–20.

2

ON RICIN AND ABRIN: QUANTITATION ENTERS IMMUNITY RESEARCH

I have here the possibility ... to deal with the question of immunity in a more mathematical manner.

Paul Ehrlich, 1891

WHY WORK ON PLANT TOXINS?

We must go back for a moment to June 1890 when Ehrlich, in his private laboratory, commenced experiments on the plant toxins ricin and abrin.[1] Since it was these experiments that caused him to enter the young field of immunology (not yet so-named), it may be valuable to explore the reasons for this apparent departure from his more usual research pursuits in histology, hematology, and the clinical problems encountered in his daily practice.

The view in the 1880s of the causes of disease was quite different from that existing today. For some thousands of years, it was generally believed that disease was caused by poisons arising from the slimes and miasms of unhealthy places. Indeed, the Latin word for poison was *virus,* and it is no coincidence that Louis Pasteur, who identified microorganisms as the etiological agents of disease, called these organisms *virus.* Even the words *virulence,* now used to denote the degree of danger posed by a pathogen, once measured the poisonousness of a substance. Indeed, the words *pharmacy* and *pharmacopoiea* are derived from the Greek equivalent word, and refer to both a helpful drug or a harmful poison.

Then, in 1888, Emile Roux and Alexandre Yersin discovered the toxin associated with the diphtheria organism,[2] and it was quickly demonstrated that the disease is caused by the toxin alone, rather than by the direct action of the microorganism itself. Shortly thereafter, Shibasaburo Kitasato in Koch's laboratory at the Hygienic Institute in Berlin performed the same service with respect to tetanus, showing that it is an exotoxin elaborated by the *Clostridium* that causes the disease.[3] Along similar lines, as we saw in Chapter 1, Robert Koch thought that his tuberculin was an analogous toxic product of the tubercle bacillus.[4] These recent demonstrations appeared to lend strong support to the classical theory that all infectious diseases are caused by toxins elaborated by the organisms involved.

Thus, in early 1890, toxins as disease agents were very much in the air in Berlin, as elsewhere. In addition, because the medical research community in Berlin was modest in size, it is likely that Paul Ehrlich, even working apart in his private laboratory, would have heard by early summer of 1890 of the startling results from the Hygienic Institute across town. There, Behring and Kitasato were in the process of discovering substances in the blood of immunized animals that would protect normal animals from the deadly effects of diphtheria and tetanus toxins; they would not publish these results until December.[5] There also, Robert Koch was preparing his long-awaited announcement of a possible cure of the dreaded tuberculosis. He would propose using the putative toxin tuberculin to counter the disease, just as Louis Pasteur had employed chicken cholera and anthrax organisms to combat these diseases by altering the susceptibility of the host itself (i.e., by inducing immunity).

The stage was now set for the imaginative Paul Ehrlich, steeped in structural chemistry, partial to quantitative methods, and with the seeds of a comprehensive theory of biological interactions already at hand, to tackle the problem of the mechanisms of immunity to toxins. He was, after all, generally interested in the pathogenesis of disease, and had previously studied the toxic effects of such substances as iodine, phosphorus, and cocaine. That Ehrlich was aware of the significance of poisons in disease pathogenesis is made clear by the opening sentences with which he introduced his ricin studies:

> In the course of my investigations on the relationship which exists for a vast number of substances between chemical constitution, the distribution within individual organs, and physiological activity, as was quite obvious from systematic experiments, I was also led necessarily to the meaningful study of poisonous proteins. When I report the results obtained herein, it was done especially for the reason that I believe that from many points of view this same relationship ought to be of interest for an understanding of infectious diseases.[6]

Furthermore, Ehrlich appeared to be confident that he could introduce quantitative chemical science into research on immunity, as he had introduced these methods in the fields of histology, hematology, and cellular physiology. Since the toxic bacterial proteins such as diphtheria and tetanus toxins have not yet been produced in pure state or in commercial quantities, he proposed to study the readily available and pure ricin, derived from the castor bean, and abrin, obtained from the jequirity bean.

RICIN STUDIES

The Experimental System

Ehrlich commences the study in his typical style; he looks for a suitable experimental animal and establishes the reproducibility of the approach. He finds that 1 g of the commercial ricin is sufficient to kill one and one-half million guinea pigs, and marvels that it is many thousandfold more toxic than the better known poisons mercuric chloride and cyanide. Although standard laboratory white mice are less sensitive to ricin than guinea pigs, Ehrlich is able to show that a reproducible titration curve of ricin toxicity may be established in mice. The endpoint for this assay is measured in terms of the dilution of a standard solution of ricin that causes death in a 20-g animal within 2 to 4 days. He feels justified then in concluding that, "I have here the possibility ... to deal with the question of immunity in *a more mathematical manner* (Ehrlich's italics).[7]

But, for ricin, the normal mode of immunization via the subcutaneous route proves too damaging because severe local inflammation with induration and scarring makes further study difficult. It is here that Ehrlich's technical inventiveness comes effectively into play.[8] He finds that feeding of the toxin will also permit quantitative assay of toxicity, but without deleterious side effects that would interfere with further experimentation. He then devises a reproducible feeding method, involving the addition of the desired amount of a solution of toxin to a biscuit (the so-called *Albertcake*) to form a stiff dough. This is then divided into small cubes (aliquots), dried, and fed to the mouse, assuring a known dosage. The technique became quite popular, and was called *die Ehrlich'sche Cakesmethode.* Preliminary tests showed that by this route, 0.02 mg of ricin is tolerated, whereas 0.035 mg is the median dose (MLD) causing death in 5 to 6 days.[9]

Immunity to Ricin

Now Ehrlich is ready to demonstrate the induction of immunity in mice (Table 2.1). He starts with an oral dose of 0.002 mg (or roughly 1/17 the MLD) and increases the dosage slowly. Already after day 11, he is able to administer a lethal dose with impunity, and by the eighth week the animal is able to tolerate more

TABLE 2.1   Introduction of Stepwise *per os* Immunization

Day	Lethal doses	Day	Lethal doses	Day	Lethal doses
1[a]	0.06	19	3.1	41	12.3
3	0.11	21	3.4	42	(severe diarrhea)
5	0.22	23	4.0		
7	0.33	25	4.6	43	8.0 (recovered)
9	0.43	29	6.0	45	8.6
11	0.86	31	6.8	48	10.0
13	1.4	34	8.6	51	11
14	1.7	37	10.6	53	12
16	2.3	39	11.4	54	14 (weight loss)

Source: Adapted from the first table in the ricin paper (*Collected Papers,* vol. II, p. 23).

[a] I have only included every other entry. Day 1 was 10 June, 1890.

TABLE 2.2   The Time-Course of the Immune Response

Day	Largest dose fed (μg)	No. of animals	Maximum dose tolerated (MLDs)	Observations
4	4	8	<1	All >1 MLD dead
5	5	16	1.3	Minor necrosis
6	6	23	13.3	Extensive necrosis
7	7	5	10	Minor necrosis
8	8	18	20	Miniml necrosis
10	12	9	40	Negligible necrosis
12	20	3	66.6	Mild necrosis
15	50	1	100	—
18	80	4	200	Massive necrosis
21	80	1	400	Necrosis of the abdominal region

Source: Adapted from the second table in the ricin paper (*Collected Papers* vol. II p. 24).

than 10 MLDs. He decides not to carry the process further, since the animal is refusing to feed and losing weight. He finds that the slow increase to about 3 MLDs as the maximum immunizing dose *per os* suffices to yield adequate protection, and that any additional increase in the level of immunity may better be attained by using the subcutaneous route.

Already at this time, Ehrlich was measuring the level of immunity in numerical terms (*Immunitätsgraden* = degree of immunity). This was the measure of the greatest number of lethal doses that the immunized animal could resist. He points out that levels of immunity up to 200 can be attained readily with the feeding protocol; higher degrees of immunity (up to 800) may be reached only with an additional series of systematically increasing subcutaneous doses. To demonstrate the time-course of the development of immunity and to obviate individual differences among mice, Ehrlich has run six different experimental series, involving many animals. Here, the maximum tolerated subcutaneous challenge dose is titrated at different times after initiation of the feeding protocol, as illustrated in Table 2.2.

It can be seen from this table that during the first 5 days of immunization, there is no significant protection afforded. Suddenly, on the sixth day, a very obvious immunity has appeared, rendering the animals resistant to over 13 lethal doses, although the immunity is not perfect as indicated by the development of some necrosis at the challenge site. Ever imaginative in search of clinical correlates of his results, Ehrlich says,

> The most noteworthy finding that surprised me most is the sudden—I might say critical—appearance of immunity on the sixth day. One automatically is led to the speculation that the critical fall of the fevers in so many diseases, as in pneumonia and measles, which frequently occurs at the end of the first week, *is attributable to a similar event, the critical onset of immunity* [Ehrlich's italics].[10]

Thenceforth, the immunity continues to increase in progressive fashion, reaching a value of 400 by the end of the third week; by feeding he has never been able to exceed a degree of immunity greater than 1000. He points out that if the results are graphed, a curve in the shape of a parabola is obtained, wherein the degree of immunity attained approaches an asymptote. He is able to show further that small doses (e.g., 3 µg per feeding) administered over prolonged periods may elicit levels of immunity as high as the large dose regimen, reaching 200 after 7 weeks *and then going no higher.* He points out further that per unit of toxin employed, the immune response is greater using low doses than high, one of the earliest suggestions that there is no one-to-one relationship between immunizing agent and the substance responsible for protection.[11]

The Duration of Immunity

Ehrlich next proposes to ascertain whether immunity is only a temporary property or instead a long-lasting acquisition of the organism. He therefore progressively immunizes a group of mice (he calls them *"ricinisirt"*) to a minimal titer of 200, and is able to show persisting high immunity on challenge at 6 $^1/_2$ and 7 $^1/_2$ months. He states that he intends to study this phenomenon more extensively to establish the duration of immunity difinitively. Ehrlich mentions the "fundamentally important discovery" of diphtheria and tetanus antitoxins by Behring and Kitasato and that they have shown by passive transfer of protection to normal animals that immunity is carried in the blood. He then furnishes an analogous demonstration that in the ricin system, the protective substance (which he terms "antiricin") also resides in the blood of immunized animals, both mouse and rabbit. He further shows that the duration of this passive immunity in the recipient is related to the protective titer of the blood donor. Although Ehrlich has not yet established the precise duration of what will become known as passive immunity, it appears to last a much shorter time than does active immunity.

Ophthalmic Studies

The imaginative Ehrlich is not content merely to demonstrate the toxicity of ricin at subcutaneous and gastrointestinal locations, and the protection afforded at these sites following immunization. He goes on to demonstrate ricin toxicity in the eye upon conjunctival application, and that the protection that follows systemic immunization involves the eye also. Even a thick paste of ricin applied to the eye of an immune animal elicits no toxic response. As Ehrlich says, "It is a question here in the eye also of *an absolute immunity of a local type,* which seems to be developed even at moderate levels of general resistance to ricin." This mention of ocular immunity is the earliest harbinger of an interest that will be taken up by ophthalmologists with the ultimate development of a full subdiscipline, that of ocular immunology.[12] Ehrlich will expand on the significance of this ocular immunity in the abrin studies described next.

ABRIN STUDIES

Having demonstrated in his ricin studies the technique for the induction of high degrees of antitoxic immunity, and the way that the level of immunity may be measured quantitatively, Ehrlich now extends these results to another plant toxin, abrin.[13] But it soon becomes apparent that he is not interested in the simple repetition of the same type of result merely to justify another publication (an approach not entirely unknown in recent times!); he already knows that these data can be generalized to diphtheria and tetanus toxins. Rather, he has two other important points to make with the abrin studies. He will utilize the immune response to prove that ricin and abrin are *different* toxins, and show no antigenic cross-reaction. He will also discuss the significance of local ocular immunity, in that it may permit the use of abrin therapeutically for the treatment of trachoma. First, however, Ehrlich methodically demonstrates that the immunization protocol developed for ricin applies equally to abrin, and that similar protective anti-abrin titers can be achieved (although abrin appears to have only about one-seventh the toxicity of ricin when fed).[14] He demonstrates both systemic immunity to subcutaneous challenge and ocular immunity to conjunctival application of the toxin. As with ricin, Ehrlich is able to conclude for abrin that *"All of these features are based, as may readily be demonstrated, upon the presence in the blood of a body—anti-abrin—which paralyzes the activity of abrin, apparently by the destruction of these [toxic] substances"* [his italics].[15]

Immunological Specificity

Ehrlich pays tribute to the extensive studies of ricin and abrin by Kobert and his colleagues at the Physiological Institute in Dorpat, who have brought these toxins to the attention of the medical community and the products themselves to commercial availability.[16] Both are proteins susceptible to the action of proteolytic enzymes, and both produce substantially similar physiological effects (although abrin causes extensive hair loss, whereas ricin does not). Thus, despite some difference in their intrinsic toxicities, it is still not fully clear that they are in fact different substances.

Ehrlich proposes, therefore, to answer the question of the relationship between the two plant toxins immunologically. After demonstrating the resistance to ricin of ricin-immune animals, he shows that both systemically and locally in the eye there is no resistance to abrin; abrin evokes as great an inflammatory reaction in ricin-immune animals as in normal controls. Similarly, abrin-immune animals show no greater resistance to the action of ricin than do normal animals. There is no cross-protection to be seen. With his usual incisive logic, Ehrlich concludes,

> It would be scarcely imaginable to propose a more striking proof that antiabrin and antiricin have no relationship to one-another. It follows also from this that the otherwise so similar starting materials which cause the production of two different antibodies are themselves completely different [his italics].[17]

This is the first time the nature of immunological specificity has been so well understood that it could be applied to the qualitative analysis of antigens.

Implications for Ocular Therapy

In the 1880s, ophthalmologists were interested in the therapeutic use of plant toxins such as abrin to clear up certain corneal lesions, and especially the corneal inflammation caused by trachoma. There had been a report from Brazil by the Belgian ophthalmologist L. de Wecker entitled "Experimental purulent ophthalmitis produced by means of jequirity or licorice vine."[18] de Wecker tested abrin for the treatment of trachoma, but decided against its use due to the severe conjunctival inflammation that accompanied its instillation on the eye. Ehrlich's awareness of this report demonstrates yet again Ehrlich's encyclopedic knowledge of the literature in so many diverse fields.

Among the ricin experiments that Ehrlich repeated using abrin was the demonstration that abrin-immune animals can also resist abrin's toxic effects on the conjunctiva. He pointed out, therefore, that the danger of using abrin topically to heal corneal ulcers can be obviated by systemic preimmunization with abrin, thus permitting its use in clinical practice. But Ehrlich went further. He showed the potential clinical importance of his observations in that, commencing with the conjunctival instillation in *normal* animals of very low doses with cautious daily increase in dose, inflammation might be avoided without compromising abrin's therapeutic effect. He ends the discussion with very precise advice on the proper dosages, timing, and cautions to be observed in the treatment of human patients. This was the first demonstration of the ability to immunize via the conjunctival route and of the presumed local formation of antibodies in the eye, a phenomenon that was to prove highly important in future studies of ocular immunology.[19]

Further Studies

At the end of the abrin paper, Ehrlich mentions that he has performed experiments similar to those previously mentioned with a third plant toxin robin, derived from the bark of the acacia. A weaker toxin than either ricin or abrin, robin nevertheless was able to induce immunity just as readily as these two. In a later publication, Ehrlich discussed experiments from his laboratory by Morgenroth on yet another plant toxin crotin, which yielded similar results.[20]

Mechanism of Action of Toxins

In his paper "On the constitution of toxins" in the *Ehrlich Festschrift,*[21] Hans Aronson pointed out that it had been suggested by Roux and Buchner that antitoxin acts indirectly by modifying the host's ability to be damaged. Ehrlich countered this argument by taking advantage of the fact that ricin is able *in vitro* to agglutinate erythrocytes. He mixed varying amounts of antiricin serum with highly toxic ricin, and could demonstrate that antiricin neutralizes the agglutinating activity of ricin *in vitro* precisely in parallel with its protective power *in vivo*.[22] This had to be by direct chemical interaction of antitoxin with toxin, quite in line with all of Ehrlich's previous views of biological interactions. Not long thereafter, Ehrlich's colleague Morgenroth would confirm this conclusion elegantly by demonstrating the *in vitro* neutralization of the enzyme rennin by antirennin.[23]

SIGNIFICANCE OF THE WORK

For the near term, Ehrlich's results had a marked impact on immunological thinking and practice. First, he demonstrated that protective immunity is not limited to bacterial toxins; even plant toxins, to which humans are normally not exposed, may stimulate an immune response. This must perforce have affected any view that the immune response is a *direct and specific* Darwinian adaptation to the threat of the common dangerous pathogens.[24] By the end of the 1890s, the issue was further clouded by the finding that the immune response could respond to a wide variety of *bland* antigens, and even to cells of the body!

Next, Ehrlich's demonstration that high titers of antiserum may be obtained by starting with low initial amounts of antigen, with progressive increases in dosage; this approach set the tone for all future immunization protocols. This was especially true for such toxins as diphtheria and tetanus, whose popularity in the new serotherapy grew steadily. Only with the development of toxoids and active immunization of humans would new protocols be introduced, involving far fewer injections and greater doses. Implicit also in this phase of the work was the fact that small amounts of antigen might give rise to large amounts of antibody, arguing strongly against the direct conversion of the one to the other.

Ehrlich's finding that actively induced immunity was long-lasting implied either that the *Körper* (bodies) responsible for neutralization of the toxin persist in the blood of the immunized animal or that the process of their formation continues after cessation of the immunizing injections. But these same antibodies disappear moderately rapidly when transferred to normal recipients, suggesting that it is the latter alternative that applies.

The parallel decrease in the activity of toxin in its *in vitro* and *in vivo* manifestations when antitoxin is added made it clear that it is not the susceptibility of the host on which the antitoxin acts. Rather, it would thereafter be generally understood that the antibody acts directly on the antigen, either to neutralize it or to destroy it.

Perhaps the most generally interesting of Ehrlich's speculations about these studies follows from his surprise at the sudden onset of immunity on the 6th day of immunization. Could an active response to the infectious agent, heretofore considered only as a preventive measure, be responsible for an abrupt change in symptomatolgy? Such a possibility would have important implications for the understanding of the natural history of such disease processes. It is curious that Ehrlich specifically mentions measles in this context. He is speaking here about the 6th day *after the onset of symptoms,* and suggests that it is the immune response that ends the symptoms. A decade later, 29-year-old pediatric resident Clemens von Pirquet would claim for measles and similar diseases that it is the development of immunity that *initiates* the disease symtoms.[25] Thus, the end of the rash and fever is not the beginning of pathogen clearance, but its completion! This view has been confirmed in modern times, with the demonstration that these symptoms result from the action of cytotoxic T cells functioning to clear the virus from infected cells in the skin and elsewhere.[26] In the immunocompromised host, the rash and fever are substantially absent; measles presents as a giant cell pneumonia.[27]

Ehrlich's suggestion that local ocular immunity might render abrin treatment of trachoma more tolerable apparently did not convert the ophthalmic community, for reasons that are not clear. However, his demonstration of immunity in ocular tissues did intrigue many ophthalmologists. They then initiated a variety of experiments in the eyes of laboratory animals, and began to interpret a variety of ocular diseases in immunological terms; this led eventually to the development of organized research in ocular immunology and immunopathology, eventually with all the characteristics of an established discipline.[28]

Finally, perhaps the most significant result of Ehrlich's studies of plant toxins was to convince him that immunity research was not a trivial pursuit, but rather one worthy of his future full-time attention.

A NOTE ON ORAL IMMUNIZATION

In the course of assembling the Ehrlich bibliography (Appendix), I ran across his brief note on the history of immunization *per os.*[29] Others had apparently claimed priority for the approach and Ehrlich, typically, was quick to contest any challenge to his own achievements and priorities. But the exchange called to mind contemporary confusion associated with oral administration of antigen.

With the discovery of the mucosal immune system, involving secretory IgA and its importance in diseases of the gastrointestinal and upper respiratory tracts, interest in oral immunization has swelled. This was heralded by the introduction of an oral poliomyelitis vaccine, and the hope of attaining an efficacious oral cholera vaccine. The oral administration of other preventive vaccines, including genetically modified carriers, is currently under consideration and even testing.[30] But from another direction come conflicting reports—oral administration of certain immunogens may apparently lead to a state of *immunological tolerance* rather than to positive immunity.[31] This approach has been favored by many in the field of autoimmune diseases, who employ "self" antigens in an attempt to prevent or alleviate autoimmune diseases. However, it is not evident that there are substantial differences, either qualitative or quantitative, in the protocols employed by the immunizers on the one hand, or the tolerizers on the other. Indeed, the induction of an autoimmune disease following oral administration of autoantigen has been reported.[32] We will eagerly look forward to the future resolution of this paradox.

NOTES AND REFERENCES

1. Ehrlich's studies of the immunology of plant toxins are discussed at length in several chapters in the *Ehrlich Festschrift:* Th. Madsen, "Method and quantitative principles in dealing with problems of immunity," pp. 151–158; Hans Aronson, "The constitution of toxins," pp. 166–190; and H. Ritz, "Plant toxins," pp. 200–208.
2. Roux, E. and Yersin, A., *Ann. Inst. Pasteur* 2:629, 1888.
3. Kitasato, S., *Allg. Wien. med. Zeitung,* 34:221, 1889; *Deutsch. med. Wochenschr.* 15:635, 1889.
4. Koch, R., *Deutsch, med. Wochenschr.* 16:1029, 1890.
5. Behring E. and Kitasato, S., *Deutsch. med. Wochenschr.* 16:1113, 1890. See also Behring, ibid. 16:1145, 1890.
6. Ehrlich, P., *Deutsch, med. Wochenschr.* 17:976, 1891; *Collected Papers* vol. II, pp. 21–26.
7. Ehrlich, note 6, *Collecte Papers,* vol. II, p. 22.
8. See Marks, L.H., *Ehrlich Festschrift,* pp. 159–161. Marks details many instances of Ehrlich's novel experimental designs and innovations and uses the ricin feeding method of immunization as one of the chief examples.
9. Ehrlich is not always clear on the precise dosages used in these studies, sometimes expressing doses in dilutions of the toxin in saline (e.g., 1:200,00) where the volume is not always stated, sometimes in milligrams of toxin per animal. In the table on p. 24 of the ricin paper in vol. II of *Collected Papers,* apparently the column labeled "milligrams" should be "micrograms"! I have reworked the numbers as best I could understand the text.
10. Ehrlich, note 6, *Collected Papers* vol. II, p. 25.
11. This implication of Ehrlich's results was apparently not recognized by Hans Buchner who in 1893 (*Münch. med. Wochenschr.* 40:449, 480, 482) suggested that antitoxin is formed directly from the toxin itself by some fairly simple transformation.
12. The birth of this new discipline of ocular immunology is discussed in Silverstein, A.M., *Cell. Immunol.* **136,** 504, 1991.
13. Ehrlich, P., *Deutsch, med. Wochenschr.* 17:1218, 1891; *Collected Papers* vol. II, pp. 27–30.
14. Ehrlich speculates on whether this represents an intrinsic difference in toxicity, or merely a difference in the absorption of the two through the gut wall.
15. Ehrlich, note 13, *Collected Papers,* vol. II, p. 29.
16. Kobert, R. and Stillmark, H., *Arbeiten des Dorpater pharmakologischen Instituts,* vol. VIII, Stuttgart, Ferdinand Enke, 1889.
17. Ehrlich, note 13, *Collected Papers,* vol. II, p. 30.
18. de Wecker, L., *C.R. Acad. Sci. Paris* 95:299, 1882.
19. One of the early ophthalmic immunologists, Paul Römer, wrote a lengthy review of abrin immunity and abrin therapy, *Graefes Archiv f. Ophthalmologie* 52:72, 1901.
20. Ehrlich, P., *Berlin klin. Wochenschr.* 35:273, 1898.
21. Aronson, H., *Ehrlich Festschrift,* pp. 166–190.
22. Ehrlich, P., *Fortschr. der Medizin* 15:41, 1897; *Collected Papers* vol. II, pp. 84–85.
23. Morgenroth, J., *Centralbl. Bakt.* 26:349, 1899.
24. Elie Metchnikoff had, of course, advanced a Darwinian theory based on phagocytes (best explained in his *Immunity in the Infectious Diseases,* New York, Macmillan, reprinted by Johnson Reprint, New York, 1968). However, this process was essentially nonspecific and could not explain the origin of specific antibodies. Some modern immunologists continue to suggest that the germline genes for antibody production have been selected to protect against the most common pathogens (see, e.g., Cohn, M., Langman, R., and Geckeler, W., *Progr. Immunol.* 4:153, 1980).

25. Interestingly, Pirquet made this startling claim in a sealed letter deposited in 1903 with the Academy of Sciences in Vienna to establish his priority claim. The letter was opened and read before the Academy only in 1908; see Wagner, R., *Clemens von Pirquet: His Life and Work,* Baltimore, Johns Hopkins Press, 1968, pp. 52–55. For a discussion of Pirquet's important contributions to immunology between 1903 and 1910, see Silverstein, A.M., *Nature Immunol.* 1:453, 2000.
26. See Griffin, D.E. in ter Meulen, V. and Billeter, M.A., eds., *Measles Virus,* New York, Springer, 1995, pp. 117–134.
27. Mitus, A., Enders, J.F. *et al., N. Eng. J. Med.* 261:882, 1959; Markowitz, L.E., Chandler, F.W. *et al., J. Infect. Dis.* 158:480, 1988.
28. See Silverstein, note 12.
29. Ehrlich, P., *Wien. klin. Wschr.* 21:652, 1908.
30. McGhee, J.R. and Kiyono H., "The Mucosal Immune System" in Paul, W.E., ed., *Fundamental Immunology,* 4th ed., Philadelphia, Lippincott-Raven, 1999, pp. 909–945, especially p. 929ff.
31. See Ethan Schevach's chapter "Organ-specific Autoimmunity" in Paul, W.E., ed., *Fundamental Immunology,* 4th ed., Philadelphia, Lippincott-Raven, 1999, pp. 1089–1125, especially p. 1118 ff.
32. Blanas, E. *et al., Science* 274:1707, 1996.

3

THE VALUE OF
MOTHER'S MILK:
THE FOUNDING OF
PEDIATRIC IMMUNOLOGY

I have been able to succeed in finding a simple research plan...
Paul Ehrlich, 1892

Most immunologists will recognize the name Paul Ehrlich as one of the Nobel Prize-winning founders of their discipline, with his quantitative assay of diphtheria toxin and antitoxin, his side-chain theory of antibody formation, and his elegant studies of immune hemolysis. But few if any immunologists, and no pediatricians whom I have questioned, are aware that Ehrlich performed the first critical experiments in pediatric immunology. He demonstrated the manner in which the fetus and neonate acquire protective immunity from the mother and stressed the importance of milk antibodies. His contributions to this field are scarcely mentioned in definitive works on the subject, such as *The Transmission of Passive Immunity from Mother to Young*[1] or *Maternofoetal Transmission of Immunoglobulins.*[2] and not at all in more general summaries, for example, *Foetal and Neonatal Immunology*[3] or *Immunology and Immunopathology of the Human Foetal-Maternal Interaction.*[4] To have forgotten Ehrlich's contributions is especially surprising, since these animal experiments may be classed not only as among the most elegant of all of those devised by this imaginative investigator, but as ranking high also among *all* 19th-century experimental designs.[5]

BACKGROUND TO THE STUDIES

Why should Ehrlich have become interested in the immunological relationship between mother and offspring in 1892, the year after his introduction to immunology through his work on abrin and ricin? Nothing in his writings provides a clear answer, but we may make a reasonable inference from an understanding of the contemporary state of knowledge and Ehrlich's approach to science. He wanted always to understand the *why* of things and processes, and to theorize about their origins and mode of function. He was well aware of the then-mysterious mechanisms of natural and acquired immunity through the famous works of Pasteur, Koch, and Metchnikoff. Further, the great stir in the medical community and beyond that followed the discovery of diphtheria and tetanus antitoxins by Behring and Kitasato[6] meant that physicians everywhere were alert to signs of immunity to these diseases. Thus, Ehrlich must have been familiar with the frequent reports that newborn children may be initially resistant to the diphtheria bacillus and often show protective blood titers of diphtheria antitoxin. An omnivorous reader of the entire medical literature, he also was aware of the many reports indicating that young animals may inherit from their parents protection against a variety of other infectious diseases.

We saw in the preceding chapter that Ehrlich's venture into immunity research not only produced valuable data, but appeared also to stimulate him to consider questions about the basic mechanisms of antibody origin and function. Given the success of the ricin-abrin experiments, we may surmise that Ehrlich felt that the solution of the problem of the inheritance of immunity might lead to an explanation of the mystery of the origin of protective antibodies. As he says in the introduction to his major study of the bases of neonatal immunity,[7]

> One of the most important tasks in medicine lies in the solution of the problem of how the organism can protect itself against infections. ... In the light of our current ideas and understanding, the Jennerian discovery no longer appears to be an inexplicable and isolated phenomenon, but rather as the expression of a fundamental principle which dominates the majority and perhaps the entirety of infectious diseases—that of immunity.[8]

ORIGIN OF IMMUNITY IN FETUS AND NEONATE

Ehrlich published the results of his initial studies in 1892, in a paper entitled "On immunity by inheritance and suckling." Referring in his introduction to the earlier, often conflicting, reports of neonatal protection, he concluded,

> Thus I believe that I can assert that these essentially incidental observations do not provide an explanation of *the so-called nature of inheritance, insofar as three different possibilities present themselves which, differing in principle, must also be separately treated. The immunity of the offspring can be effected by: 1) inheritance in the ontogenetic sense; 2) the transfer of maternal antibody; and 3) the direct intrauterine influence on the fetal tissues by the immunizing agent.* ... I have been able to succeed in finding a simple research plan which made it possible to establish in each instance the mechanism of inherited immunity [his italics].[9]

Here is Ehrlich at his most typical. The elegance of this "simple research plan" will quickly become apparent.

Is Immunity Inherited Genetically?

First, Ehrlich planned what he called an *experimentum crucis,* to test whether neonatal immunity is derived from the father or mother. At that time, it was commonly believed that certain diseases and even immunity might be transmitted from the father[10] and even from the grandfather[11] by way of an "altered zygote." These experiments were based on Ehrlich's earlier demonstration that a dependable "absolute lethal dose" of the plant toxins ricin and abrin can be established for mice of a standard weight.[12] Thus, partial immunity in the test animals is made evident by an extended survival time as compared with controls, and greater levels of protection result in less severe lesions or none at all.

Ehrlich first tested the offspring of immune fathers and normal mothers and found that they showed no protection; doses in the range of 0.2 to 1.3 lethal doses routinely produced severe lesions up to death within 4 days. By contrast, the offspring of normal fathers and immune mothers were almost routinely protected, even against multiples of the lethal dose. Table 3.1 illustrates not only the protection afforded the newborn by its immune mother, but in addition the duration of this immunity. It can be seen that the neonate enjoyed almost complete protection from these toxins for about the first 6 weeks postpartum. The immunity then waned over the succeeding few weeks, and had completely disappeared by the third month of life.

TABLE 3.1   Immunity to Ricin or Abrin in the Newborn of Immune Mothers and Normal Fathers

Age (days)	Toxin	No. of lethal doses	Result
21	Abrin	0.66	Normal
21	"	1.33	"
21	"	1.33	"
35	Ricin	5.00	"
42	"	10.00	Extensive necrosis
46	"	4.00	Normal
56	Abrin	4.00	Necrosis, + day 14
61	"	0.33	Hair loss, necrosis
61	"	1.33	+ day 4
69	"	1.10	"
81	"	0.25	"
81	"	1.33	"
87	Ricin	2.00	+ day 5
92	"	1.00	Intense induration
97	"	1.60	+ day 3
97	Abrin	1.25	+ day 4
102	"	1.00	+ day 5

Source: Adapted from Ehrlich, note 7, Table II, *Collected Papers,* vol. II, p. 34.

Further experiments along these same lines, but now using the offspring of nonimmune parents derived from ricin- or abrin-immune grandparents, showed that immunity to these toxins was never transmitted to the second generation. He could conclude, therefore, that immunity was carried neither by an "altered zygote" nor by paternal sperm. Following the lead provided by Behring and Kitasato's demonstration of serotherapy using diphtheria antitoxin, Ehrlich summarized this phase of the study,

> We can presently distinguish two types of immunity, the first of which may be termed active and the second passive. ... It is not to be doubted that the immunity *that we have observed in the offspring of immune mothers ... depends on the transfer of maternal antibody* [his italics].[13]

The Foster-Mother Experiments

But Ehrlich did not yet know how and when antibody is transferred from mother to offspring. The starting point was the observation that the immunity derived from passively administered antibody disappears much more rapidly in the adult mouse than does that derived by the newborn from its mother. This meant to Ehrlich either (a) that the newborn conserves passive antibody better than the adult does,[14] or (b) that a new external source develops. The latter can only be from the milk. Therefore, Ehrlich devised a lovely set of experiments to decide the question, whose difficulty can only be appreciated by those who have tried similar studies: the transfer of newborn mice from their natural mothers to suckle on foster mothers.[15]

Ehrlich transferred the neonates prior to suckling from their abrin-immune mother mice to nonimmune foster mothers. As Table 3.2 shows, these mice initially had modest levels of anti-abrin immunity that rapidly disappeared; this immunity

TABLE 3.2   Newborn Mouse Exchange Experiment—Abrin System

Abrin-immune wetnurse (suckling newborns of nonimmune mothers)			Normal wetnurse (suckling newborns of abrin-immune mothers)		
Age (days)	Challenge (lethal doses)	Result	Age (days)	Challenge (lethal doses)	Result
27	1.25	Normal	22	1.25	Necrosis
29	3.33	± induration	24	3.33	+ day 5
31	10.00	± induration			
37	40.00	+ day 5			
(Wetnurse survived 40 lethal doses)			(Wetnurse + day 5 after 1.25 lethal doses)		

Source: Adapted from Ehrlich, note 7, Table IV, *Collected Papers,* p. 38.

TABLE 3.3   Newborn Mouse Exchange Experiment—Ricin System

Ricin-immune wetnurse (suckling newborns of nonimmune mothers)			Normal wetnurse (suckling newborns of ricin-immune mothers)		
Age (days)	Challenge (lethal doses)	Result	Age (days)	Challenge (lethal doses)	Result
20	2.25	Normal	20	2.25	± necrosis
21	10.00	"	21	10.00	+ day 5
23	20.00	Induration	23	5.00	Severe induration
25	13.33	3+ induration	25	13.33	+ day 2
27	40.00	Severe necrosis			
41	2.00	3+ necrosis + day 12			

Source: Adapted from Ehrlich, note 7, Table V, Collected papers, p. 39.

could only have been acquired passively *in utero*. (Ehrlich was never able to show that antigen derived from the mother during gestation could stimulate an active immune response in the fetus.) By contrast, the offspring of nonimmune mothers transferred to immune wetnurses demonstrated high levels of anti-abrin protection that lasted for some weeks after weaning. So effective was this passive immunity derived from the milk that at its height the neonate was found to resist more than 10 lethal doses of toxin. A repeat of these newborn exchange experiments using the ricin system provided further confirmation of these results (Table 3.3). Once again, the offspring of a ricin-immune mother given to suckle to a nonimmune wetnurse showed a degree of immunity that lasted for some 3 weeks. The results obtained with normal offspring that suckled from an immune wetnurse were even more convincing; immunity lasted at least 6 weeks, and at its peak substantially protected against over 40 lethal doses. Ehrlich could now conclude,

> From this experiment it is shown with certainty—as was to be expected *a priori*—that the young come into the world endowed with maternal antibody ... that already after 21 days the degree of immunity is extraordinarily low. ... On the other hand ... my experiments show with every certainty that milk ... supplies antibody to the suckling young and provides a high and increasing immunity throughout the duration of suckling.[16]

Ehrlich then raised the question of the origin of milk antibodies. Is this due to a restricted change in the function of the mammary gland or is antibody formation a normal function of this tissue? The solution was extraordinarily simple. In a preview of future experiments, he transfered horse anti-tetanus serum (obtained "from my good friend Kitasato") passively to a nonimmune nursing mother, and demonstrated the appearance of complete immunity in the suckling young within the next 24 hours. He points out that, until now, blood was considered to be the only carrier of protective antibodies. That the milk also may contain antibody is readily understandable, since the mammary gland is the only one that secretes large quantities of protein.

Ehrlich next discussed the curious and hitherto unknown fact that the antibodies in question appear to pass unchanged through the intestinal wall of the newborn into its circulation. As he put it,

> More wonderful, however, is the fact that the antitoxins suckled with the milk can enter the circulation from the alimentary canal unaltered. We are accustomed to view antibodies as extraordinarily labile substances. … It is thus a phenomenon worthy of note that in this instance the antibodies contained in the milk are not subjected to decomposition and destruction by the potent action of digestive juices. This process is even more unusual, since I have never succeeded in detecting the slightest trace of antibody by feeding [normal animals] with pieces of the organs of highly immune animals.[17]

Clinical Implications

Then, always interested in the practical, Ehrlich began a long discussion of the clinical implications of his findings. He suggested that he has now established that it is maternal antibodies in the milk that explain why certain infectious diseases of children do not afflict suckling infants during the first year of life. As he concluded, *"Thus, mothers milk is the most ideal food for the newborn."*

Follow-up Studies

It is typical of Ehrlich that, once he had published a set of scientific findings, he would alertly scan the literature as well for confirmation of his results (which he welcomed) as for contradictions (to which he was generally quick to respond). Thus, two years later, Ehrlich published a paper with Hübener[18] that was in essence a response to several challenges to his maternal–fetal/neonatal data previously outlined. These were studies by Charrin and Gley from France[19] and Tizzoni and Centanni from Italy.[20] Both reports suggested that Ehrlich had been wrong, and that in fact immunity could be conferred to the neonate by the father. Ehrlich and Hübener's paper not only pointed out the technical errors in these two studies, but further demonstrated the validity of his earlier results. They extended these same findings to the tetanus system and to a new species, using suckling guinea pigs as well as mice. In an extensive study of the persistence of immunity in newborn mice, they were able to show clearly once again that protection against challenge by pathogenic tetanus organisms is only afforded by immune mothers and not by immune fathers; that protection continues so long as the neonate suckles from the immune mother; and that protection diminishes during the month after weaning and is completely gone by the end of the second month.

THE ORIGIN OF MILK ANTIBODIES

The results previously outlined on the importance of milk antibodies prompted further experiments on their origin. These were reported in two follow-up papers that Ehrlich published in collaboration with Ludwig Brieger, whom Robert Koch had named head of the Clinical Department at his newly formed Institute for Infectious Diseases. The experiments now shifted to the goat, from which much greater amounts of milk could be obtained. In their first paper,[21] they immunized a pregnant goat with increasing doses of a dilute tetanus toxin about 5 weeks prior to parturition. During the second month of the injection series, they shifted to a more virulent culture fluid, and showed that the animal could ultimately tolerate at least 80 lethal doses of the toxin without ill effects. Within 24 hours following birth of the kid, protective antibodies appeared in the milk.

They then set up a quantitative assay of the protective power of the milk. They pointed out that there are two approaches to the titration of protective antibody. The first, favored by Behring in his studies of diphtheria antitoxin,[22] measures the dilution of the antitoxic fluid required to neutralize a certain toxic effect. The second approach measures the number of units of toxin (lethal doses) that are required to just overcome the protective effect of a given amount of the antitoxic fluid. Brieger and Ehrlich choose this second approach, although they confess that with careful technique both should yield identical results.

They employ a standard toxic preparation of tetanus bouillon whose lethal dose for a standard mouse had previously been determined. They then titrate the antibody content of the milk as follows: a given volume of milk is injected into a series of mice, which are then challenged with increasing doses of tetanus. The number of lethal doses tolerated by the mice is determined, and the titer is expressed as immunity units/cc milk/g of mouse. Table 3.4 illustrates a typical titration of the antibodies found in goat's milk on the 41st day of immunization (i.e., 1 week after birth. They conclude that this volume of milk protects the 20-g mouse against some 16 to 24 lethal doses, for a titer of between 1600 and 2400 units (i.e., 16 lethal doses × 20 grams × 1/0.2 cc milk

TABLE 3.4   Titration of the Tetanus Antitoxin Content of Goat's Milk (0.2 cc. of Milk Administered Intraperitoneally)

Animal number	No. lethal doses	Result
1	4	Normal
2	8	Normal
3	16	Transient mild disease
4	20	+ day 5
5	24	Disease day 2 with recovery
6	32	+ day 2
7	40	+ day 2
8	48	+ day 2

Source: Adapted from Brieger and Ehrlich, note 21, second table, *Collected Papers* vol. II, p. 46.

= 1600 immunity units/gram of mouse/cc of milk). Here was the approach that Ehrlich would elaborate in his famous 1897 demonstration of how to measure the potency of diphtheria toxin and antitoxin.[23]

Brieger and Ehrlich note that they were unable to elicit protection by feeding immune goat's milk to adult mice. They point out, however, that in the fetus the antibodies *(Schützkörper)* pass freely and promptly from the intestines to the circulation. It will, they say, be their task to clarify the basis for this difference between the neonatal and adult intestinal tracts. Finally, Brieger and Ehrlich point out that milk may provide a most useful source for the isolation of these protective substances. They conclude their first paper by reporting that removal of the casein leaves the original protective capacity untouched, and that vacuum evaporation of the residual whey substantially concentrates the active factor.

In their second paper on milk antibodies,[24] Brieger and Ehrlich exploit the goat's milk system in two directions: first, to elucidate the dynamics of the immune response and, next, to show in detail how antibodies may readily be obtained in quantity from milk. They point out that the goat is the most appropriate animal for these studies and that tetanus is the best system because it is the best example of a pure toxic disease, and also because its endpoint is clearest.

THE DYNAMICS OF THE IMMUNE RESPONSE

Brieger and Ehrlich introduce this study by recalling that appreciable quantities of antibody are present in the milk of an immunized, lactating goat after 41 days. They indicate that the further aim is to determine (1) whether the excretion of these antibodies lasts throughout the entire period of lactation and (2) if, this being the case, the antibody content of the milk increases with the rise in immunity of the animal.

As in Ehrlich's earlier work with ricin and abrin, Brieger and he use steadily increasing doses of antigen to immunize their lactating goats in the present study.[25] Moreover, they measure the antibody content of the milk every few days, permitting them to plot a curve of the kinetics of the antibody response. This approach depends on the assumption that the milk titer reflects absolutely the changing titer in the blood, an assumption apparently justified by the earlier observation that passive antibody administered to a nursing mouse is rapidly reflected in the suckling newborn. This means that the normal mammary gland contributes little to the active formation of antibody.[26]

The authors then describe the changes in titer resulting from subsequent (booster) injections of antigen. This plots as a curve that they describe as a "waveform" (Fig. 3.1), in which an immune animal with some 4000 units of antibody suffers an initial decline in titer during the next 2 days to almost 1000 units. The titer then rapidly rises over the next 17 days to a peak of almost 9000 units, before falling somewhat during the following weeks.[27] Figure 3.2 shows that each additional antigenic boost yields a similar waveform, and each one leads to a higher titer of protective antibody.

THOUSANDS

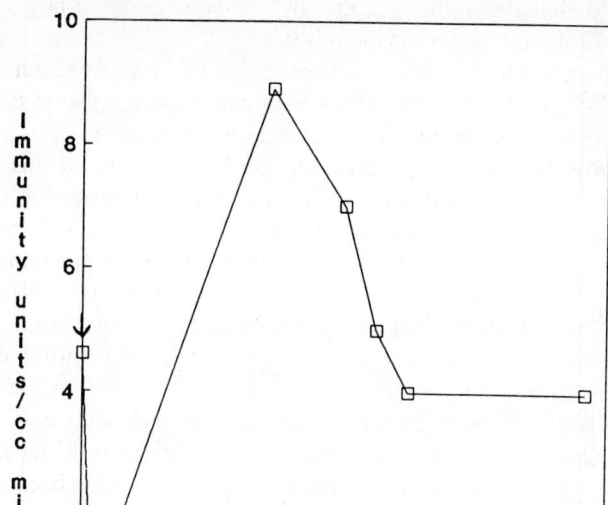

FIGURE 3.1   Dynamics of the antibody response measured in the milk of a lactating goat after a single booster injection of tetanus toxin. (After Brieger and Ehrlich, note 24.)

The authors conclude that "such types of curve hint at a complicated biological state of affairs."[28] They then analyze the significance of each phase of the immune response curve in terms that are some 40 to 50 years ahead of their time. Phase I, the fall: the large amount of antigen in the booster injection "directly binding or otherwise destroying the existing antibody in the immunized animal, leading to a corresponding reduction in the amount secreted in the milk." This would later be shown to accompany the immune elimination of antigen.[29] Phase II, the rise: this is due to the active response of the host, involving an overproduction or overcompensation for the earlier fall in titer. (Note this anticipation of Ehrlich's later side-chain theory of antibody formation—the same words are employed.) Phase III, the reduced steady state: the host now attains a [slowly declining] steady state until the next booster immunization intervenes.

Brieger and Ehrlich point out the practical significance of the several portions of the antibody response curve. First, it shows the importance of repeated booster injections. Next, it emphasizes the critical nature of the timing of bleeding of the immunized animal in order to obtain therapeutic antisera. It should be done at the

THOUSANDS

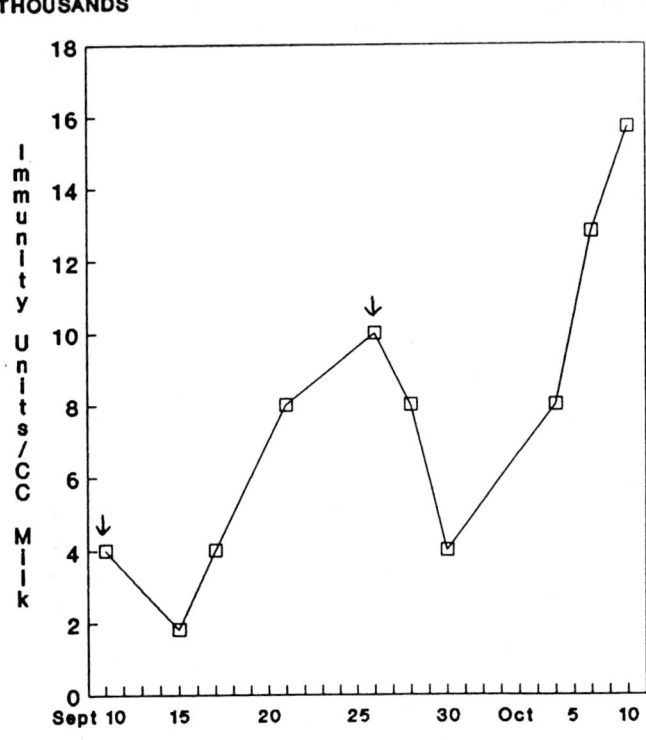

1892

FIGURE 3.2   Dynamics of the antibody response of the lactating goat to repeated booster injections of tetanus toxin. The injections are indicated by arrows. (After Brieger and Ehrlichm, note 24.)

peak of the booster response; too early, during the immune elimination phase leads to low titers, as does bleeding too late during the phase of declining concentrations of antibody.

THE PURIFICATION OF MILK ANTIBODY

Brieger and Ehrlich then moved on to the next major experiments—the purification of antibody from milk. They report immediately that "We have now found that in a single step one can isolate substances of considerable protective value from milk and other protein-rich fluids."[30] After trying a large variety of precipitating agents, including acids, alcohols, and metal salts, by far the best results were obtained with ammonium sulfate. The antibody precipitates in the first fraction, at 27–30% ammonium sulfate, leaving much protein behind.[31] The material is then dissolved in water, dialysed, and evaporated in vacuum, yielding a powder readily soluble in water. With concentration comes an increase in potency, so that milk with a titer of 2000 to 6500 immunity units yielded a powder with a titer of 900,000 to 4,000,000, or a concentration factor of 400–600. They pointed out that concentrating antibody from serum is not as efficient, since there are so many other proteins that coprecipitate with the antibodies. Similar findings were obtained later by Ehrlich and Wassermann for the diphtheria toxin-antitoxin system.[32]

DISCUSSION

Here is a series of groundbreaking and even elegant studies by a remarkable scientist. Far in advance of his time, Ehrlich and his colleagues contributed important information for our understanding of some of the most basic aspects of immunology. As nearly as I can determine, he was the first to clearly define the difference between active and passive immunity. He was surely the first to interpret the basis for neonatal protection against many infectious diseases, demonstrating transplacental transfer of maternal antibodies and then the role of milk-borne antibodies in protecting the neonate. This early demonstration of the dynamics of the antibody response illustrated well the phase of immune elimination of antigen (reflected in a transient reduction in blood/milk titer) and then the heightened titer that follows the booster injection of antigen. A similar understanding of the characteristics of the immune response would not reappear until the 1950s.[33] The fact that these kinetics were immediately reflected in the antibody titers in the milk showed that these antibodies originate from the blood.

It is of interest that Ehrlich mentions Darwin in connection with these studies. This is, surprisingly, the only reference to Darwin that I have found in any of Ehrlich's papers, despite the obvious Darwinian nature of many of his ideas and especially of his later side-chain theory. In discussing his proposed tests of paternal transmission of immunity, he points out that "It will generally be agreed, in contrast to *the original Darwinian theory,* that acquired characteristics are not inherited as such" [my italics].[34] But certain cases of congenital malformation recall the question. "Thus the possibility cannot be excluded that such striking modifications of a special organ part may be readily inherited (and immunity represents such a modification of the entire organism)." It is to test this possible inheritance of an acquired characteristic that Ehrlich has designed his *experimentum crucis.*

Curiously, these studies of the transmission of immunity to the offspring constitute almost the only instance in which Ehrlich's scientific activities failed to exert a lasting effect on biomedical science. It is true that in the years immediately after these publications, they appeared to stimulate a number of follow-up studies, but these were done as often to contradict as to confirm and extend Ehrlich's results. Thereafter, the work appears to have been substantially forgotten, and the burst of research activity on maternal–fetal/newborn immunological relationships in the period after World War II (1–4) seems to have received its impetus from other sources.

This important work deserves to be better known.[35]

NOTES AND REFERENCES

1. Brambell, F.W.R., *The Transmission of Passive Immunity from Mother to Young,* Amsterdam, North Holland, 1970.
2. Hemmings, W.A., ed. *Maternofoetal Transmission of Immunoglobulins,* Cambridge, Cambridge University Press, 1976.
3. Solomon, J.B., *Foetal and Neonatal Immunology,* Amsterdam, North Holland, 1971.
4. Loke, Y.W., *Immunology and Immunopathology of the Human Foetal-Maternal Interaction,* Amsterdam, North Holland, 1978.
5. I have also pointed out the elegance of these experiments in *Nature Immunol.* 1:93, 2000.
6. Behring, E. and Kitasato, S., *Deutsch. med. Wochenschr.* 16:1113, 1890.
7. Ehrlich, P., *Z. Hyg. Infektkr.* 12:183, 1892; *Collected Papers,* vol. II, pp. 31–44.
8. Ehrlich, note 6, *Collected Papers,* vol. II, p. 31.
9. Ehrlich, note 6, *Collected Papers,* vol. II, pp. 31–32.
10. Ehrlich quotes Arloing, S., *Les Virus,* Paris, Alcan, 1891, p. 285: "When the father is cured of a virulent disease, when he participates in the act of fertilization, he can moreover transmit a portion of the immunity which he enjoys. The male sperm, origin of the fertilizing capacity, has been dynamically modified at the end of the father's disease … it carries into the ovum during penetration a vaccinated substance which is distributed in all of the cells of the fetus and embryo." See also Fournier, A. (known to contemporaries as "le pape des syphiligraphes"), *L'Hérédité Syphilitique,* Paris, Masson, 1891.
11. Fournier, E., *Hérédo-syphilis de Seconde Génération,* Paris, Rueff, 1905.
12. The "absolute lethal dose" is one that kills all 20-g mice in 2–4 days. Hoever, more sensitive animals may succumb during this period to as little as one-fourth this amount.
13. Ehrlich, note 7, *Collected Papers,* vol. II, p. 35.
14. Ehrlich was not aware that heterologous proteins are cleared from the circulation much more rapidly than homologous ones, due to immune elimination of antigen through the formation of immune complexes. His passive transfer studies employed rabbit anti-ricin in the adult mouse, whereas the newborn mouse received maternal mouse antibodies. Only some 60 years later would this distinction become widely known: Talmage, D.W., Dixon, F.J., Bukantz, S.C., and Dammin, G.J., *J. Immunol.* **67,** 243, 1951; Dixon, F.J., *J. Allergy* **25,** 487, 1954.
15. These experimenta are difficult because lactating female mice will generally reject (and often kill) newborns not their own.
16. Ehrlich, note 6, *Collected Papers,* vol. II, pp. 39–40.
17. Ehrlich, note 6, *Collected Papers* vol. II, p. 41.
18. Ehrlich, P. and Hübener, W., *Deutsch. med. Wochenschr.* 18:51, 1894; *Collected Papers,* vol. II, pp. 63–71.
19. Charrin, A. and Gley, E., *Arch. Physiol.* 4:75, 1893; idem, *Arch. Physiol.* 6:1, 1894.
20. Tizzoni, G. and Centanni, E., *Riforma Med. Napoli* 9:101, 1893; idem, *Centralbl. Bakt. Parasit.* 13:81, 1893.
21. Brieger, L. and Ehrlich, P., *Deutsch. med. Wochenschr.* 18:393, 1892.; *Collected Papers,* vol. II, pp. 45–47.
22. See, e.g., Behring, E. and Frank, *Deutsch. med. Wochenschr.* 18:348, 1892; also Schütz, *Z. Hyg. Infektionskr.* 12:58, 1892.
23. Ehrlich, P., *Klin. Jahrb.* 6:299, 1897/8; *Collected Papers* vol. II, pp. 86–106.
24. Brieger, L. and Ehrlich, P., *Z. Hyg. Infektkr.* 13:336, 1893; *Collected Papers,* vol. II, pp. 48–55.
25. In a footnote to this article signed by Ehrlich alone (*Collected papers,* vol. II, p. 49), he objects to Behring's claim that the method of immunization employing steadily increasing doses of toxin is his own intellectual property (Behring, E., *Die Blutserumtherapie,* vol. I, Leipzig, Thieme Verlag, 1892. As always, Ehrlich is quick to defend his claims to scientific priority.
26. Sixty years later, an elegant series of experiments by Ita Askonas and coworkers (*Biochem J.* 56:597, 1954) would confirm and extend Brieger and Ehrlich's findings, and show that most antibody in rabbit's milk and in goat's colostrum and milk is a transudate from the blood, without

degradation and reformation. However, the presence of plasma cells within the mammary gland, especially after local immunization, demonstrates that local antibody formation is also possible.

27. Brieger and Ehrlich, note 24, point out in a footnote that Emil Behring had independently reported similar findings in his recently published book *Die Blutserumtherapie,* (note 25), vol. II, p. 108.

28. Brieger and Ehrlich, note 24, *Collected Papers,* vol. II, p. 51.

29. Clemens von Pirquet would later point to this fall in circulating antigen as due to the formation of the immune complexes which cause serum sickness (*Allergy,* Chicago, American Medical Association, 1911). See Silverstein, A.M., *Nature Immunology* 1:453, 2000.

30. Brieger and Ehrlich, note 24, *Collected Papers,* vol. II, p. 54.

31. Until the advent of preparative electrophoresis, ion exchange columns, and especially of monoclonal antibody technics, several generations of immunologists would utilize this ammonium sulfate approach for the concentration of immunoglobulins.

32. Ehrlich, P. and Wassermann, A., *Z. Hyg. Infektkr.* 18:239, 1894; *Collected Papers,* vol. II, pp. 72–79.

33. In an elegant study of the primary and anamnestic response employing radioiodine-labeled antigens, F.J. Dixon, P.H. Maurer, and M.P. Deichmiller (*J. Immunol.* 72:179, 1954) published substantially the same wave-shaped curves illustrating the phases of the immune response that Ehrlich had presented in 1892 (see Figs. 1 and 2), but apparently were unaware of this earlier work.

34. It is not generally remembered that in his original formulation, Darwin did allow for a certain amount of "soft" inheritance. See Ernst Mayr's Prologue to *The Evolutionary Synthesis,* E. Mayr and W.B. Provine, eds., Cambridge, Harvard University Press, 1980, pp. 1–48.

35. To illustrate how little remembered was this pediatric work of Ehrlich, I have mentioned elsewhere (*A History of Immunology,* New York, Academic Press, 1989, p. xi) that one of the principal reasons for my entry into the history of immunology was the receipt in the mid-1970s of a paper to review, written by a young scientist who was unaware that he had repeated work done 80 years earlier by Paul Ehrlich. That work was his study of the origin of passive immunity in the suckling young.

4

THE STANDARDIZATION
OF TOXINS AND
ANTITOXINS

*Ehrlich's immunity unit plays the same role for antitoxin
measurement as does the Standard Meter for the measurement
of length.*

Thorvald Madsen, 1914

The demonstration in 1890 by Emil Behring and Shibasaburo Kitasato[1] that immunization with a toxin results in the formation of a blood-borne protective substance excited the medical world. Not only did it suggest a humoralist explanation for the immunity that follows Jennerian vaccination for smallpox and Pasteurian immunization for anthrax and rabies,[2] but it offered much more. The immunized host was not only protected from diphtheria or tetanus, but its blood could be transferred passively to protect naive recipients or even to cure the disease once started. There was, in the circulation of immunized individuals, some sort of protective "body." At a time when the pathogenesis of infectious diseases was thought to involve the action of poisons (toxins) liberated by the pathogen,[3] Behring and Kitasato's discovery was widely viewed as the key to the eventual cure of all these diseases. Thus, before it appeared that the approach was limited to only those few pathogens that liberate exotoxins, and that passive transfer of xenogeneic serum might cause serum sickness, Behring would be awarded the first Nobel Prize for Medicine in 1901, and would be ennobled by the Kaiser.

The initial attempts to prepare diphtheria antitoxic sera and treat infected children clinically met with widely varied success. Different donor animal species were employed, the dosages of antitoxic serum employed could not be standardized, and little attention was paid to the progress and severity of the disease in the patient. Thus, varying and conflicting reports of the efficacy of diphtheria antitoxin in the cure of childhood diphtheria appeared in the literature,[4] and physicians throughout the world often employed serum preparations containing little or no protective antibody.[5] Indeed, even Behring and the Hoechst Company (with whom Behring had a joint arrangement for the production and sale of diphtheria antitoxic serum) were having difficulty in producing a high-titer product, and the Hoechst directors were starting to complain about the cost of the project.[6]

Ehrlich's Rational Approach

Having already demonstrated with ricin and abrin how high titers of antitoxic sera can be produced *and measured* (see Chapters 2 and 3), Ehrlich turned his attention to the quantitative aspects of diphtheria antitoxin production, assay, and clinical application. By this time he was well established in Robert Koch's Institute for Infectious Diseases and widely recognized for his careful and quantitative experimentation. It was only the direct request of Behring, urged on by an impatient Koch and a cost-conscious Hoechst Company, that would allow Ehrlich to venture into an area to which his institute colleague had full priority claim. The fact that August Wassermann collaborated in Ehrlich's first publication in this field was significant, a further indication of Director Koch's support of Ehrlich's involvement in this important new therapeutic approach.

Ehrlich's first paper on the subject, published in 1894 with Kossel and Wassermann, was entitled "On the Production and Use of Diphtheria Antiserum."[7] Ehrlich was careful in the introduction to pay tribute to Behring's original discovery, and indeed mentioned that the investigations here reported "have been undertaken in agreement with Behring, and with the warmest interest and authoritative advice of our highly honored chief, Herrn Geheimrat R. Koch." He also mentions that the studies have extended over several years (so that they must have begun already in 1892), not surprising in view of the impressive amount of data included in the five pages of the report. Ehrlich would bring to the study of diphtheria toxin and its antitoxin the same careful quantitative approach that he had employed with ricin and abrin.

First, they will use goats as antiserum producers; not only did this species serve well in the ricin and abrin studies, but preliminary results showed that these animals are highly sensitive to dipheria toxin and also produce very high titers of antitoxic antibody. In addition, the demonstrated ability to prepare large quantities of antibody from goat's milk may also be important for these studies. They report that high titers of antitoxin may also be produced also in the cow.

The second point that they emphasize is the importance of obtaining high titers of antibody, on the resonable assumption that the more antibody used, the greater the clinical efficacy of the treatment. For this, they revert to Ehrlich's earlier demonstration with ricin that repeated injections with increasing doses of toxin will result in higher and higher titers. They will therefore start to immunize with increasing doses of a killed culture of bacilli to obtain a "basic immunity," and then shift to increasing doses of the most virulent cultures of living bacteria available, to maximize the immune response.

Since the ultimate purpose of the investigation is the practical value of the method for treating diphtheria in humans, the authors point out the critical importance of having an accurate and reproducible assay of the antitoxic activity of their sera. Until then, the usual method for the titration of antitoxic sera was to inject a given amount into test animals (usually guinea pigs) and then determine how much injected toxin that dose would protect against. But because the reaction must occur *within the test animal,* it is too slow and too dependent on individual variation in the resorption of the reagents, yielding results that are too variable. Rather, the authors will take advantage of the original observation in Behring and Kitasato's first report that antitoxin will neutralize toxin *in vitro.* They will therefore measure the antitoxin content of their sera by premixing in the test tube varying amounts of serum with a standard preparation of toxin. The resulting mixture is then injected into the guinea pig to test for residual toxicity. This approach is permitted, they claim, because they have shown that the *in vitro* combination is rapid and "obeys the simple law of proportionality." Here is a method that assures a rapid, quantitative, and reproducible result.[8] With this approach, they define one "Immunization Unit" (IE) as the mount of antiserum required to neutralize 1.0 cc of Behrings standard toxin, or 0.8 cc of their more potent preparation.

The Clinical Trial

Ehrlich and his coworkers will now, "in agreement with Prof. Behring," employ their highest titer antitoxin preparations in the treatment of diphtheritic children in a number of different Berlin hospitals. With the aid of the directors and staff of six different Berlin Institutions, they have been able to treat a total of 220 cases of childhood diphtheria. (In addition, they are able to control their treatment regimen by comparing their cases with comparable groups of untreated diphtheritic children.)

They start initially with single injections of serum containing 130–200 units of antitoxin, but later in more severe cases utilize repeated injections of the antitoxic serum to increase the dosage. Of the total cases treated with antitoxin, 168 of the 220 recovered, or 76.4%; the remainder died. Of the 220 treated children, 67 had already been given a tracheotomy, and the success rate in this group was only 55.1% (We may assume that only the most severe cases with the worse prognosis were tracheotomized—those whose breathing had been impaired by the development of diphtheritic membranes.)

When the data were analyzed further, they were able to show for the first time the importance of the timing of treatment after onset of disease. The survival rate was 100% when antitoxin treatment was started on the first day of symptoms, 97% on day 2; 86% on day 3; 77% on day 4; and 56% on day 5. Thus, when serotherapy is begun within the first 2 days, only 2/72 patients died, whereas 25/72 untreated controls died. They point out that many of the cases that serotherapy failed to save had come to them too late and had suffered from intercurrent infections; conversely, they feel that with sufficient antitoxin administered early enough, they could probably have saved at least half of the children lost.

The conclusions drawn from these studies for the first time provide serotherapy with a rational basis:

1. The fate of the child is determined in the first 3 days of disease; serotherapy should commence as early as possible.
2. Since a surplus of antitoxin in the body of the child should be attained, mild cases should be given at least 200 immunization units, and severe cases and all tracheotomized cases at least 400 units.
3. Serum treatment should be repeated on the same day or on subsequent days, depending on the course of fever, pulse, and local factors. The total amount of antitoxin may reach 500 to as many as 1500 units according to the severity of the case.
4. The authors caution, however, that these results apply only to *their* sera, and that other preparations must be assayed and have values equal to theirs to be equally affective.

In order to gain a wider audience for the successful serotherapeutic trials, Ehrlich and Kossel summarize the study in a subsequent paper entitled "On the Use of Diphtheria Antitoxin."[9] They again emphasize the critical importance of employing high titer antisera, multiple doses, and early treatment. There is an extensive discussion of clinical matters, including the prognosis of serious cases requiring tracheotomy, and of the complications of diphtheria, including accompanying bacterial infections and organ failure. They have, in effect, provided in two pages a *vade mecum* for the clinician facing an outbreak of diphtheria.

ANTITOXIN FROM SERUM AND MILK

Some months after the demonstration of the efficacy of diphtheria serotherapy, Ehrlich and Wassermann published a paper on the isolation of diphtheria antitoxin from serum and milk.[10] In their preliminary study on a single goat, begun in 1892,[11] they confirm the earlier results obtained with ricin: the goat readily makes diphtheria antitoxin; the protective substance appears in the milk; and milk titers of antitoxin parallel those in the serum. Thus, they feel justified in extending the study to many additional animals, while repeating the emphasis on the importance of using progressively higher doses of antigen to assure high titers.

To underline the importance of having a good assay method for antitoxin, Ehrlich and Wassermann reexamine the two approaches to the titration of antitoxins. They show that the method of premixing toxin and antitoxin *in vitro* is much more sensitive than passively immunizing the guinea pig and then challenging with toxin. In addition, the endpoint is more precise. Thus, utilizing a standard toxin, the difference between a severe reaction and none at all in the *in vitro* test is from 0.005 to 0.006 cc, or 20%, whereas the same difference in the *in vivo* approach is from 0.024 to 0.060 cc, or 150% However, as they show in detailed titrations using constant antiserum and variable toxin, there is a certain variability among the guinea pigs available for the test.

They next compare the antitetanus and antidiphtheria toxin titers of milk and serum of immunized goats, and demonstrate that serum contains some 15 to 30 times (usually about 20 times) as much antibody as milk whey. Despite the lesser concentration of antitoxin in the milk as compared with the blood, they point out that one may obtain a liter of milk per day from the lactating goat, or 30 liters per month. This would have the same antitoxin content as 1.5 liters of blood, an amount greater that the goat could provide without serious consequences. With concentration of the whey therefore, as shown in the earlier publication with Brieger,[12] an even more effective preparation of protective antitoxin should be available from milk than from blood.[13] Once again, the authors state that, in conjunction with Professor Behring, they will utilise the highest titer sera available to test further their practical therapeutic use in various Berlin hospitals.

Ehrlich then gave a lecture before the German Society for Public Health Care.[14] He reviews briefly the history of the discovery of the diphtheria bacillus, its toxin, and specific diphtheria antitoxin. He emphasizes the importance of accurate assays of these reagents, and describes how it became apparent that only high-titer antisera are maximally effective in therapy. He then summarizes his own involvement in this area, first with the plant toxins ricin and abrin, then with the production of high-titer antisera and preparations derived from milk, and finally with the clinical application of these sera in the treatment of diphtheria in children.

It would appear that the chief purpose of the lecture is to reassure practitioners that serum therapy is not only efficacious, but safe as well. He discusses the previous clinical studies involving the use of passively administered diphtheria antitoxic serum and concludes that it causes no untoward side effects; any later nephritis or myocarditis that may be encountered is due, he claims, to the direct effect of the diphtheria toxin on these organs.[15]

The impressive immunological studies that Ehrlich had reported on plant toxins, on the maternal–fetal relationship, and on diphtheria antitoxin, came to the attention of Ministerial Director Friedrich Althoff at the Prussian Ministry of Education. It was apparent to all that Ehrlich held the key to the solution of the practical problems involved in diphtheria serotherapy, and Althoff arranged for Ehrlich to become head of a Royal Institute for Serumtesting and Serum Research in Berlin-Steglitz.[16] It was a modest establishment, but it was his own, and it represented the first official recognition of his scientific worth. From this laboratory would come, during the next few years, some of Ehrlich's most interesting contributions to the developing field of immunology.

THE MECHANISM OF ANTITOXIN ACTION

Ehrlich's first report from his new institute was entitled "On the knowledge of the action of antitoxin."[17] In it, he reviewed current theories of the action of antibody. Behring had initially supposed that the antitoxin directly destroys the toxin molecule, but this was soon shown to be an incorrect assumption. Roux and Vaillard[18] had shown that mixtures of toxin and antitoxin harmless to normal animals were still toxic in weakened animals, while Buchner[19] found that such neutral mixtures that spared the mouse would kill the guinea pig. Both results demonstrated that some free toxin might persist in the presence of antitoxin, and these investigators concluded that the antitoxin did not function by destroying the toxin itself. Rather, they assumed that the antitoxin protected the animal by acting directly on its tissue cells to protect them from the poison.

But perhaps the best indication that the toxin molecule survives the action of antitoxin was the finding with snake toxins. Calmette[20] and, independently, Physalix and Bertrand[21] had shown that an antitoxin could be produced against the toxins of the naja and the cobra. Calmette then reported that when inactive combinations of a snake toxin and its specific antitoxin were heated, the thermolabile antitoxin is destroyed, restoring the toxicity of the thermostable toxin.[22] In light of these observations, Ehrlich suggests two possibilities to explain the action of antitoxin: first, that Roux and Buchner are correct in thinking that the antitoxin acts on the target cell, making it insensitive to the effect of toxin; or second, that the antibody neutralizes the toxin by combining with it, thus inhibiting its deleterious effects (a chemical view fully reflective of Ehrlich's notions about the nature of biological reactions).

Ehrlich points out that it is very difficult to obtain decisive results by experimentation using the complex *in vivo* systems, and that *in vitro* experiments, especially with pure materials such as ricin, are to be preferred. He urges acceptance of the assumption that the action of these plant toxins is directly analogous to the systems involving diphtheria or tetanus toxins, a viewpoint supported by the fact that, as he says, "his ricin studies have not been deemed unimportant in this connection,"[23] The stage is now set for the presentation of quantitative results utilizing the ricin-antiricin system and the generalization of these results to all toxin-antitoxin systems.

Ehrlich first shows that ricin will agglutinate the erythrocytes of defibrinated blood in the test tube, and that he can titer an anti-ricin by measurung its ability to interfere with the agglutination by a given quantity of ricin. Next, he demonstrates that a parallel titration of ricin and its antibody can be done *in vivo* by injecting into the mouse mixtures of antitoxin and toxin in various ratios, and evaluating the resultant degree of inflammation or death of the animal. Ehrlich concludes that, "There exists between the two experimental series [i.e., *in vivo* and *in vitro*] an absolute agreement not only in qualitative but also in quantitative relationship."[24]

Ehrlich thus concludes that these results argue against the cellular view of Roux and Buchner, in that they involve no vital process. He believes that his earlier suggestion of a purely chemical interaction is supported, and expresses the hope that further investigations will permit a closer view of the "finer chemistry" of this puzzling situation.

Ehrlich did indeed expand later on these observations, but in a manner that illustrates a sharp difference between the way that scientific communication was carried on in late 19th-century Europe and how it functions in modern society. The world of what we now call biomedical practice and research was small; many important reports were delivered at the meetings of the various medical and scientific societies and these *and the discussions that accompanied them* were widely reported in such German weekly publications as the *Berliner klinische Wochenschrift,* the *Deutsche medizinische Wochenschrift,* the *Münchener medizinische Wochenschrift,* and so on; in France in the *Comptes Rendus de la Sociéte de Biologie,* and the *Comptes Rendus de l'Academie des Sciences,* and so on; and in Britain in the *Proceedings of the Royal Society.* Many important data were presented during these somewhat informal comments that would be recorded, but might never be published formally in an appropriate journal.

Thus, following a paper read by H. Kossel at a meeting of the *Society of Charité Physicians,*[25] in which he reported a study using the toxin of eel serum, Ehrlich rose to comment.[26] After complimenting Kossel, he mentioned work on the plant toxin crotin performed by his assistant Morgenroth. In contrast to ricin, which agglutinates erythrocytes, crotin hemolyzes those of certain species, a property that can be inhibited by specific anti-crotin antiserum. Ehrlich mentions that he himself has shown that tetanus toxin is not one but two poisons; the first is the classical toxin that induces tetany (tetanospasmin), whereas the second is a substance that hemolyzes the erythrocytes of many species (tetanolysin). This second toxic substance, says Ehrlich, also engenders its own specific antitoxin. This is an important new finding to be reported so informally, and neither Morgenroth nor Ehrlich seem to have followed up these casual statements with formal publications.

It was Madsen who drew attention to these studies in his paper in the Festschrift celebrating Ehrlich's 60th birthday.[27] Madsen had come to Ehrlich's institute from Copenhagen at this time, to study and work, and was assigned to follow up the tetanus work. He stresses the importance of Ehrlich's observation on the two components of tetanus toxin, since it led to two very important observations: first, that in a mixture of toxins (antigens), one could be absorbed without affecting the other (e.g., tetanolysin is absorbed by erythrocytes, leaving tetanospasmin free); and, second, that in a mixture of two different antibodies formed in response to a single immunization, each functions independently of the other.[28] I believe that this was the first demonstration of a partial absorption involving antigens or antibodies, an approach that Ehrlich would later elegantly apply in showing that the red cells of one species might absorb partially the hemolytic antibodies prepared against a cross-reacting species.[29] This approach would figure significantly in future immunochemical studies, most notably in the work of Karl Landsteiner.[30]

THE DEFINITIVE ASSAY: EHRLICH'S IMMUNOLOGICAL MAGNUM OPUS

After seven years' work on the quantitative aspects of toxin–antitoxin interactions, Ehrlich published a paper that would define for the world the solution to the vexing problem of how to ensure the potency of diphtheria antitoxic sera.[31] This was no simple problem like the assay of ricin and antiricin, in which a chemically pure substance (ricin) could be weighed out. In this case, both diphtheria toxin and its antitoxin were labile, and the toxin solution itself usually contained substances that interfered with the assay. It was thus impossible to develop standards for the assay; one day's titration results could usually not be repeated on the morrow. As Ehrlich points out in the introduction to the paper, the failures worldwide of diphtheria serotherapy were due to the use of antisera that were too weak to be effective.[32] He concludes the introduction with the words, "It was necessary to work out *a new and more accurate method of determining the value of the serum*" [his italics].

It is clear that in order to establish a reproducible assay system, a single permanent and dependable reference standard must be established, against which all other reagents can be measured. This will be a diphtheria antitoxic serum. But Ehrlich first demonstrates that the former standard serum, supposedly stabilized in glycerine, may deteriorate with time. Just because it might yield the same results over time, when tested against a given solution of toxin, is no proof of stability; they may both deteriorate in parallel, concealing the loss of potency of the antiserum. He concludes, therefore, that the use of solutions must be avoided. Since the chief factors in the breakdown of unstable substances are (1) water (by hydration); (2) oxygen (by oxidation); (3) light; and (4) heat, he will prepare a serum standard by maintaining dessicated aliquots of a high-titer antiserum in an evacuated chamber in the dark and cold.[33] Knowing at the start the titer of this standard, one tube can be opened as needed, dissolved in an appropriate volume of glycerinated saline, and utilized for up to 1 month to assay solutions of toxin. These in turn will permit the assay of test batches of antitoxin to determine their adequacy for use in the clinical treatment of diphtheria cases. The preparation of large numbers of tubes of the standard antitoxin will thus provide not only for the long-term maintenance of the reference standard, but will also permit the distribution of the standard throughout the world, thus assuring uniformity of reagents and, ideally, the widespread use of an efficacious therapy. Obviously, when the original reference standard nears depletion, it can be used in the preparation of a further large number of ampoules of a new, accurately assayed and thus standardized reference anttoxic serum.

Ever the careful experimenter, Ehrlich next points out the problems involved in assessing the endpoint of a titration involving living animals. He shows that the assay of a certain degree of inflammation as an endpoint is too subjective and depends too greatly on the precise site of inoculation. Therefore, the objective endpoint of death within 4–5 days of a standard 250-g guinea pig will be used to define the unit lethal dose of a diphtheria toxin solution.

Now Ehrlich sets up a series of titrations of 11 different preparations of diphtheria toxin, both from his own laboratory and from others in Germany and abroad. He tests an arbitrarily chosen standard diphtheria antiserum, diluted to contain one "immunity unit" (defined as the amount of antitoxin required to neutralize 100 lethal doses of toxin), against varying dilutions of the test toxins, and seeks to define two threshhold values: L_0, or the amount of toxin just neutralized by one unit of antitoxin, and L_+, the amount of toxin that will suffice to leave one lethal dose of toxin free after the unit of antitoxin has exerted its neutralizing effect. As Ehrlich points out, $L_+ - L_0$ should equal one lethal dose (i.e., L_0 should equal 100 and L_+ should equal 101 lethal doses) "provided the toxin *is a pure chemical substance.*"

But in no instance does reality accord with theory. Among the 11 toxin preparations tested, the values of L_0 range from a low of 27.5 to a high of 108, and for L_+, from 29 to 123. In no instance was the value of $L_+ - L_0$ equal to the theoretical one lethal dose; it ranged from 1.7 to as high as 22 lethal doses! How was this possible? Not only did some toxin preparations appear to contain substances that lowered the protective power of the antitoxin, other preparations seemed to contain substances that actually appeared to enhance its protective power. Here was a major challenge to the nimble imagination of Paul Ehrlich.

To explain these unusual findings, Ehrlich would recall that, some years earlier, he had had occasion to treat a tetanus broth with carbon disulfide in order to see the effect of substituting the amino groups of the tetanus toxin. He was surprised to find that while the preparation had entirely lost its toxicity, it possessed an even better capacity to induce immunity in mice than the original toxin. Indeed, the modified product, which Ehrlich named *toxoid,* demonstrated an undiminished ability to combine with its antibody, both *in vivo* and *in vitro.*[34] Here was proof that the structure on the toxin molecule responsible for toxicity, which Ehrlich named the *toxophore group,* differed from that responsible for attachment, which Ehrlich would soon call the *haptophore group* (from the Greek *aptein,* to grasp).

All these considerations were based on Ehrlich's long-time idea that such interactions were the result of the chemical binding of atomic structures, or side-chains, that fit one another like "lock and key," following the simile advanced by Emil Fischer. Suggesting that toxin and antitoxin react chemically, Ehrlich proceeded to postulate the existence of toxoids of varying combining affinity with antitoxin: some binding more strongly than normal toxin, some with equal affinity, and some with lesser affinity. In this way, by postulating mixtures of varying amounts of the several substances, he would explain why some values of L_0 and L_+ were higher and some lower than 100 lethal doses.

This approach, which Ehrlich employed to explain the complexities of toxin–antitoxin interactions, became so complicated and convoluted, and involved such disputes with other workers, as to justify a separate treatment; the factors that entered into play will be dealt with in the next chapter. It is not inappropriate to make this separation, since the correctness or incorrectness of Ehrlich's interpretation of the composition of toxin solutions in no way affects the validity of the method that he introduced for the standardization of therapeutic antisera.

Diphtheria Serotherapy and Financial Gain

This is perhaps the appropriate place to touch on an embarrassing and controversial aspect of the development of diphtheria serotherapy and the commercialization of the production, assay, and sale of the serum to the medical profession.

The event in question raised accusations of unfairness and maltreatment, and spoiled the friendship and collaboration between the two leading diphtheria serotherapy researchers, Paul Ehrlich and Emil Behring.

Following the laboratory demonstration of the efficacy of passive serotherapy in the treatment of diphtheria infection in animals and the preliminary demonstration that it might save the lives of affected children, it was clear that here was a pharmaceutical product with immense prospects. Behring had made an arrangement with the dye and pharmaceutical company Hoechst[35] that promised to net him some 10,000 marks per year against a 50–50 division of the profits. But, as noted previously, both Behring and Hoechst were experiencing great difficulty with the assay of the antiserum and they called on Ehrlich, the acknowledged authority on quantitative assays, to help solve the problem that was interfering with the commercial venture.

Initially, Behring entered into a joint agreement with Ehrlich to exploit the finished antitoxin product, whose sale would be managed by the Hoechst Company. The letter agreement that both signed in October 1893 indicated how many animals each of them should have, how the costs would be shared, and how the profits would be divided among the two of them and Hoechst.[36] So rapidly did the commercial prospects for diththeria antitoxic serum develop that in the following year a formal agreement was signed between Ehrlich and Hoechst, outlining the royalties due to Ehrlich on the sale of the antisera, either produced directly by him, or by Hoechst under his supervision.[37] The agreement was to run for 14 years and, according to Ehrlich's adoring secretary Martha Marquardt,[38] should have netted Ehrlich some 500,000 marks over this period.

While Behring was apparently not directly involved in the Ehrlich–Hoechst agreement, it undoubtedly affected his own arrangement with Hoechst. As Marquardt records, Ehrlich one day received a telegram from Hoechst, asking for an urgent meeting in the city of Halle. There he was met by Behring and a Hoechst representative. The main subject of the meeting appeared to have been Ehrlich's future plans and his oft-stated desire to have the maximum free time available for research. In the course of these conversations, Behring brought up Ehrlich's long-standing desire to have his own institute supported by the state. Behring promised, according to Marquardt, that he would exercise his weighty influence with the government to help Ehrlich to obtain this institute. But, he pointed out, as director of a state institute, Ehrlich would be ineligible to receive profits from the commercial sale of antitoxin, and thus he should withdraw from the Hoechst contract; this same consideration would not apply to Behring, who then held a professorship at Marburg University. At the same time, the Hoechst representative spoke of the double burden on the company of supporting both investigators.

Ehrlich resigned his share of the contract, but the institute promised by Behring was not forthcoming.[39] Ehrlich felt that he had been ill used by Behring, especially in view of the fact that during the first year of sales of the antiserum, Behring's share was over 350,000 marks, and in the 20 years through 1914, Behring received almost 1,850,000 marks[40] and built a veritable castle on the heights overlooking Marburg.

Ehrlich complained again and again about this treatment in subsequent years, and especially refused Behring's attempt to have Ehrlich's new institute in Frankfurt serve as the routine assay laboratory for the Behring/Hoechst products.[41] It is curious that the full story of Ehrlich's entry and withdrawal from the contract with Hoechst is not recounted either in the Bäumler biography (Bäumler had been a vice-president of Hoechst),[42] in the history of the discovery, development, and marketing of diphtheria antisera,[43] or in the biography of Emil Behring.[44]

Thus was Ehrlich's friendship for Behring terminated, never again to be fully renewed. It is telling that at Ehrlich's funeral in 1915, attended by many high notables, the already ailing Behring spoke the following words,

> Now you are at rest, dear friend…
>
> You always had a sensitive soul…
>
> And if we have hurt you … forgive us![45]

DISCUSSION

In his 1914 review of Ehrlich's quantitative approach to immunology Madsen, by then one of the world's leading diphtheria-therapy experts, pointed out that, "Ehrlich's method of measurement [of toxin and antitoxin] is the common property of all civilized nations," and "Ehrlich's immunity unit plays the same role for antitoxin measurement as does the Standard Meter for the measurement of length."[46] Topley and Wilson summarize the benefits derived from diphtheria serotherapy in their *The Principles of Bacteriology and Immunity* of 1938 by describing the fall in the case mortality rate for the [British] Metropolitan Asylums Board hospitals. In 1889, the year before Behring and Kitasato's discovery, the case-mortality rate was 40.7%; by 1896, just before Ehrlich showed how to standardize anti-diphtheria sera, it had already dropped to 21.2%. Thereafter, the rate continued to decline, falling below 10% for the first time in 1903, and then slowly declining to below 5% by the mid-1920s.[47]

After World War I, the standardization of diphtheria antisera, following Ehrlich's methods, was taken over by the Biological Standardization Commission of the League of Nations, working with selected Institutes throughout the world.[48] Several modifications of the standardization procedure were subsequently introduced, including Römer's intradermal test, which permitted multiple tests of inflammatory responses on the same animal without an endpoint of death,[49] and Ramon's demonstration that a suitable titration endpoint of toxin and antitoxin was the onset of flocculation of the antigen–antibody complex in the test tube.[50] The many contributions of Glenny and his coworkers during the 1920s and 1930s contributed importantly to the perfection of these techniques.[51]

For a time, active prophylactic immunization was pursued employing neutral toxin–antitoxin preparations, but several accidents involving toxicity of the mixture soon dissuaded the practice. Then, thanks in great measure to the devoted attention of Gustave Ramon,[52] impressive advances were made in the preparation of toxoids suitable for use in active prophylactic immunization to prevent diphtheria. Ultimately, the use of formolized diphtheria toxin as toxoid, adsorbed onto aluminum hydroxide or hydrated aluminum phosphate and given in two doses, has resulted in the virtual disappearance of diphtheria in the industrialized nations. The enforcement of childhood immunization, in the form of DPT (diphtheria, pertussis, and tetanus) inoculations, has substantially banished each of these diseases as significant public health concerns. These procedures were supported by application of the Schick intradermal test,[53] which permitted the clinician to assess the state of immunity in the patient and thus show whether active immunization would be required.[54]

So significant was the development of active immunization procedures against diphtheria toxin that by the 1930s, the name of Paul Ehrlich and his assay methods for diphtheria antisera were rarely remembered; indeed, the use of passive serotherapy is hardly mentioned in the 832-page treatise *Diphtheria Past and Present* by J. Graham Forbes published in 1932.[55]

NOTES AND REFERENCES

1. Behring E. and Kitasato, S., *Deutsch. med. Wochenschr.* 16:1113, 1890; Behring E. and Wernicke, E., *Deutsch. med. Wochenschr.* 12:10, 45, 1892.
2. This humoralist explanation of immunity was met with disbelief and perhaps dismay by Elie Metchnikoff and the adherents of his cellular theory of immunity. It initiated a decade-long dispute over the mechanism of immunity in which Paul Ehrlich became the chief spokesman for the humoralists, by virtue of his experiments on antibody activity and his side-chain theory of antibody formation. The many facets of the dispute are outlined in Silverstein, A.M., *Cell. Immunol.* 48:208, 1979, and in Silverstein, A.M., *A History of Immunology,* New York, Academic Press, 1989, pp. 38–58.
3. For a discussion of the prevailing view of the pathogenesis of infectious diseases, see Silverstein, *History of Immunology,* note 2, p. 2ff.
4. See the biography *Behring: Gestalt und Werk* by H. Zeiss and R. Bieling, Berlin, Bruno Schultz, 1941, p. 101 ff.
5. See Behring, E., *Die Blutserumtherapie,* Leipzig, Thieme, 1892; Throm, Carola, *Das Diphtherieserum: Ein neues Therapieprinzip, seine Entwicklung und Markteinführung,* Stuttgart, Wissenschaftliche Verlagsgesellschaft, 1995. Behring would repeatedly, in the *Deutsche medizinische Wochenschrift* of 1894, question the titers claimed for other preparations, especially the Schering Company's preparation used by Dr. Aronson. Finally, he called on Ehrlich to coauthor yet another such accusation; see Behring E. and Ehrlich, P., *Deutsch. med. Wochenschr.* 20:439, 1894.
6. See Bäumler, E., *Paul Ehrlich: Scientist for Life,* New York, Holmes and Meier, 1984, pp. 55–56. Bäumler was a vice-president of Hoechst with full access to its archives.
7. Ehrlich, P., Kossel, H., and Wassermann, A., *Deutsch. med. Wochenschr.* 20:353, 1894; reprinted in *Collected Papers of Paul Ehrlich,* London, Pergamon, 1957, pp. 56–60 (henceforth *Collected Papers*).
8. It is interesting that, in a footnote, Ehrlich suggests that the proof of the utility of his assay method is that even Behring is now using it (*Collected Papers,* vol. 2, p. 57). Ehrlich would not again make such an appeal to other authority in the field of immunology.
9. Ehrlich, P. and Kossel, H., *Z. Hyg. Infektskr.* 17:486, 1894; *Collected Papers* vol. II, pp. 61–62.

10. Ehrlich, P. and Wassermann, A., Z. Hyg. Infektskr. 18:239, 1894; Collected Papers vol. II, pp. 72–79. This paper was preceded in the journal by a paper by Wassermann alone (ibid. pp. 235–238) on a modification of the Brieger–Ehrlich procedure for concentrating diphtheria antitoxin from milk (see Chapter 3).

11. This experiment must have overlapped those of Brieger and Ehrlich on the appearance of anti-ricin in the milk of immunized animals (see Chapter 3). Since Wassermann had also appeared as junior author to Brieger (Chief of the Clinical Service at Koch's Institute for Infectious Diseases) on numerous papers during this period, his association with Ehrlich in these studies appears not to be happenstance.

12. Brieger, L. and Ehrlich, P., Z. Hyg. 13, 336, 1893; Collected Papers, vol. II, pp. 48–55.

13. It is interesting that, having made so strong a case for milk as the source of protective diphtheria antitoxin to be employed clinically, little is heard further of this approach in future publications. Serum from immunized large animals (mostly the horse in future clinical applications) is employed thenceforth. From the absence of any notice of untoward side effects from the use of milk, it may be reasonable to conclude that the shift to horse serum was based on factors of economy and convenience.

14. Paul Ehrlich, Hyg. Rundschau 4:1140, 1894; Collected Papers, vol. II, pp. 80–83.

15. Only many years later would it be shown that an immune complex-mediated glomerulonephritis may sometimes accompany the serum sickness that results from the use of large amounts of heterologous serum proteins. See, e.g., Weigle,, W.O., on the biological action of immune complexes, Advances Immunol. 1:283, 1961 and Unanue, E.R. and Dixon, F.J., on immune complex-mediated glomerulonephritis, Advances Immunol. 6:1, 1967.

16. Althoff played an important role during this era in supporting and furthering the already impressive German reputation in the biomedical sciences. He would obtain a professorship for Behring at Marburg, and would be instrumental in establishing in Frankfurt am Main the much larger Royal Institute for Experimental Therapy for Ehrlich in 1899.

17. Ehrlich, P., Fortschrit. Med. 15:41, 1897; Collected Papers vol. II, pp. 84–85.

18. Roux E. and Vaillard, L., Ann. Inst. Pasteur 7:65, 1894.

19. Buchner, H., Münch. med. Wochenschr. 40:449, 480, 1893.

20. Calmette, A., C.R. Soc. Biol. 6:120, 1894.

21. Physalix C. and Bertrand, G., C.R. Acad. Sci. 118:288, 1894.

22. Calmette, A., Ann. Inst. Pasteur 9:225, 1895.

23. Ehrlich, note 17, Collected Papers vol. 2, p. 84.

24. Ehrlich, note 17, Collected Papers vol. 2, p. 85.

25. Kossel, H., Berlin. klin. Wochenschr. 35:152, 1898.

26. Ehrlich, P., Berlin. klin. Wochenschr. 35:273, 1898.

27. Madsen, Th., Paul Ehrlich: Eine Darstellung seines wissenschaftichen Wirkens, Jena, Gustav Fischer, 1914, pp. 151–158, p. 155.

28. See Madsen, Th., Z. Hygiene 32:214, 239, 1899.

29. Ehrlich P. and Morgenroth, J., Berlin. klin. Wochenschr. 38:569, 1901; English transl. Collected Papers, vol. 2, pp. 278–297.

30. Landsteiner, K., The Specificity of Serological Reactions, New York, Dover 1962. This was a reprint of the 2nd English edition of 1945 with Landsteiner's complete bibliography; the original German version was Die Spezifität der serologischen Reaktionen, Berlin, Springer, 1933.

31. Ehrlich, P., Klin. Jahrbuch, 6:299, 1897; English transl. Collected Papers, vol. II, pp. 107–125. This paper also contained the first presentation of Ehrlich's side-chain theory of antibody formation and function.

32. Two authoritative reports on the inadequacy of available antitoxin preparations had been issued in 1896, one from England by the Lancet Special Commission (The Lancet, 2:182–195, 1896) and another by Madsen from Copenhagen (Experimentelle Undersögelser over Difterigiften, doctoral dissertation, Copenhagen, 1896).

33. Ehrlich carefully describes the process. Aliquots are dessicated over sulfuric acid and then introduced into a specially constructed glass apparatus in which further drying is effected with phosphoric anhydride; the ampoules are then sealed by flame under vacuum. Ehrlich, note 31, Collected Papers vol. 2, p. 108 ff.

34. Here, Ehrlich's memory and customary precision appear to fail him. He recalls these results from "my experiments with Dr. Benario on heredity (*Zeitschr. f. Hyg.* vol. XVIII)." But the paper referred to was published with Hübener (Ehrlich and Hübener, *Z. Hyg. Infektkr.* 18:51, 1894). Neither the experiments with carbon disulfide, nor the immunizations with treated tetanus toxin, nor even the naming of "toxoid" are mentioned in this paper. However, Ehrlich does state (p. 58) that Dr. Benario has participated in part in the experiments, and "will make a special report on the technic of immunization of experimental animals." Apparently this report by Benario never saw the light of day.

35. This company had originally been called Meister, Lucius, and Brüning, and was located in the town of Hoechst, now a suburb of Frankfurt am Main, where it still occupies a considerable industrial area. It later assumed the name Farbwerke Hoechst, and is commonly called simply Hoechst.

36. The terms of this brief agreement, signed by Ehrlich and Behring, are detailed by Bäumler in *Paul Ehrlich,* note 6, p. 56.

37. Again, the details of this contract are recorded in Bäumler, *Paul Ehrlich,* note 6, p. 58. It is assumed that this agreement superseded that between Ehrlich and Behring, although I find no record that the latter was formally terminated.

38. Marquardt, M., *Paul Ehrlich,* London, William Heinemann, 1949, p. 32.

39. Only several years later would Ehrlich be placed in charge of his own Institute for Serum Testing through the intercession of Althoff, as previously noted; see note 16.

40. See Throm, *Das Diphtherieserum,* note 5 p. 206. The equivalent value in the 1990s would be about 15–30 million Deutschmarks, or 8–16 million U.S. dollars.

41. Ehrlich reviews the entire history of his involvement with Behring in a 12-page letter to Althoff, and justifies his refusal to let Behring use the Frankfurt Institute to support his (Behring's) profitable involvement with diphtheria antisera; Ehrlich to Althoff, 1 November, 1906, Ehrlich Papers, Rockefeller Archives Center, N. Tarrytown, NY, 650 Eh 89, Box 1, Folder 1.

42. Bäumler, *Paul Ehrlich,* note 6.

43. Throm, *Das Diphtherieserum,* note 5.

44. Zeiss and Bieling, *Behring,* note 4. It must be noted, in connection with this work, that it gives little credit to Ehrlich's contributions to the diphtheria story. But this is not unexpected, since the biography was published in 1941 during the Nazi period, when the contribution of no Jewish scientist was recognized.

45. "Nun ruhest Du, Du lieber Freund ... Du hattest stets eine empfindliche Seele ... und wenn wir Dir wehgetan haben ... Verzeih!," cited by Marquardt, *Paul Ehrlich,* note 38, p. 34.

46. Madsen, note 27, p. 155.

47. Topley W.W.C. and Wilson, G.S., *The Principles of Bacteriology and Immunity,* 2nd ed., Baltimore, William Wood, 1938, p. 1086.

48. Report of the Biological Standardization Commission of the League of Nations, 1923.

49. Römer, P.H., *Z. Immunitätsf.* 3:208, 1909.

50. Ramon, G., *C.R. Soc. Biol.* 86:661, 711, 813, 1922.

51. See, e.g., Glenny A.T., *J. Hygiene* 24:301, 1925; Glenny and Okell, C.C., *J. Path. Bact.* 27:187, 1924; Glenny and Barr, M., *J. Path. Bact.* 34:131, 1931; 35:91, 1932.

52. Ramon, G., *C.R. Soc. Biol.* 89:2, 1338, 1923.

53. Michiels J. and Schick, B., *Z. Kinderheilk.* 5:255, 1913; Schick, B., *Münch. med. Wochenschr.* 60:2608, 1913; B. Schick and A. Topper, *Amer. J. Dis. Children,* 38:929, 1929.

54. A standard dose of diphtheria toxin is injected intradermally in the arm. A positive inflammatory reaction indicates that the patient has insufficient circulating antibody to prevent disease, whereas a "Schick-negative" response confirms adequate immunity.

55. Forbes, J.G., *Diphtheria Past and Present, its Aetiology, Distribution, Transmission, and Prevention,* London, John Bale Sons & Danielson, 1932.

5

THE TOXIN–ANTITOXIN REACTION: THEORY OUTPACES DATA

HENRY *Good God, woman, face the facts.*
ELEANOR *Which ones? We've got so many.*
James Goldman, filmscript, The Lion in Winter, 1968

We have, up to this point in the discussion of 19th-century immunology, dealt with theories controlled almost entirely by data. When immunization with live, attenuated pathogens was thought to deplete those trace elements critical to their growth[1] and therefor to confer immunity, the demonstration of immunity to inanimate toxins soon corrected this speculation. When immunization with toxins was thought to protect by inducing some sort of "habituation" to the toxic effects,[2] passive transfer of serum showed immunity to be mediated by an active substance, an "anti-body."[3] When it was believed for a time that antitoxins function only by acting on cells *in vivo,*[4] it was quickly found that they might also act *in vitro* to agglutinate or hemolyze erythrocytes.[5] Again, when it was speculated that antitoxin acts by destroying the toxin, it was soon shown that the toxin might be recovered from a neutral toxin–antitoxin mixture.[6] In all of Paul Ehrlich's involvement with the foregoing experiments, he had been guided by the overriding idea of molecules interacting stereochemically and specifically; this concept had repeatedly been confirmed by experiment.

Now we enter into a period in immunology when commitment to theory appeared to dominate data, often determining how the data were interpreted and even governing the planning of experiments.[7] For the first time Ehrlich, in seeking an explanation for a phenomenon, seemed to apply his ideas beyond the immediate requirements of the data. With an inexorable logic, he would construct a complicated theory of the nature of toxin–antitoxin interactions, at times adding one ad hoc hypothesis on another to maintain consistency, as new data emerged. (He would repeat this theory-to-excess again later, when he defended his concept of the nature and mode of action of complement in the hemolysis of red blood cells, as outlined in Chapter 7). When, earlier, Ehrlich had forcefully defended his data, he had usually settled the challenge fully and finally with new data; now that his theories were under attack, long drawn-out polemics became the rule and the debate was more often exhausted and given up rather than resolved.

INTRADISCIPLINARY TENSIONS AND CONFLICTS

The principal burden of this chapter will be to demonstrate not only the basic facts of toxin–antitoxin interactions, but how the disciplinary backgrounds of Ehrlich, Jules Bordet, and Svante Arrhenius determined their interpretation of the experimental data. Of course, the direction from which a scientist approaches his or her field is only one component of what we call *scientific style,* and we shall explore Ehrlich's style in all its aspects in Chapter 9. The influence of style (understood in its broadest sense) takes many different forms, and is the subject of a growing literature.[8] But it is worth pausing here to alert the reader to the extent to which the disciplinary origins of the protagonists almost imposed on them the theoretical positions that they championed. It is the background experience and even the culture of the science in which individuals are raised that often guides their choice of subject and technical approach, and even the type of speculations that they will permit themselves.[9]

In his debates with Bordet, Ehrlich took the side of the chemist to Bordet's biologist. Ehrlich argued molecules while Bordet argued processes. As Niels Jerne would point out 70 years later,[10] the field of immunology was then still divided between *cis-*and *trans-*immunologists, depending on whether their backgrounds and approaches were biological or chemical, respectively. The two groups approached many of the same problems, but in characteristically different ways; the immunobiologists worked forward from the first interaction of antigen with cell receptor, while the immunochemists worked backward from the final product, the antibody. Each group employed its own methods, the one concentrating on molecules and their structure and interactions (its journal eventually changed its name from *Immunochemistry* to *Molecular Immunology*) while the other concentrated on cellular functions and outcomes (and favored the journal *Cellular Immunology*). As Jerne said, with tongue in cheek, "The result is that the two hardly speak to one-another. Or rather, a *cis-*immunologist will sometimes speak to a *trans-*immunologist, but the latter rarely answers."

Even the language employed to describe phenomena and substances depended on disciplinary predilections—witness the different languages of Ehrlich on the one hand and of Jules Bordet on the other, in their debate on the nature of antibody. Ehrlich chose semantically charged names like *Ambozeptor* and *Komplement* that implied structure and function, whereas Bordet preferred more neutral words like *substance* and *alexine*.[11] Ernst Mayr has pointed out that early in the 20th century, a similar disparity of language and approach existed between the geneticists and the field naturalists in their view of evolution, until they were brought together in what has been termed "The Evolutionary Synthesis."[12]

The debate between Ehrlich and Arrhenius was characterized by a similar divide in conceptual framework and technique. In this case, Ehrlich was still the chemist, but the *organic* chemist, who pictured interactions in terms of the tight binding of stereochemically complementary molecules. Arrhenius, a physical chemist and founder of electrolyte theory, saw these interactions as the fairly loose association of ions *in equilibrium,* and thus would naturally take Ehrlich to task for his notion of the irreversibility of the antibody–antigen interaction. The stylistic differences that separated Ehrlich and Arrhenius are discussed in greater detail by Lewis Rubin[13] and Elisabeth Crawford.[14]

Sometimes the conceptual divide rested more on philosophical than methodological views. Mazumdar has described the continuing dispute over four generations between those who view Nature as a Leibnitzian seamless continuity *(natura non facit saltus)* and those who, with Kant, hold Nature to be discontinuous, with continuities only imposed by the human mind.[15] In each generation, and in such fields as botany, bacteriology, and blood-group genetics, one side saw continuous variation among species and genotypes, while the other side viewed these as discretely separated entities. As we examine Ehrlich's disputes with Bordet and Arrhenius, we become aware that here too, there existed these same continuity/discontinuity differences. For Ehrlich, there was no intermediate condition; an antitoxin either fixed tightly to its toxin or not at all. Ehrlich's model was the epitome of discontinuity. For Bordet and Arrhenius, however, the combination could vary continuously. Bordet would suggest the analogy of the interaction of dye with fabric, a physical adsorption that could involve continuously variable proportions of interactants. Arrhenius, on the other hand, suggested the same variability of proportions, but based now on the reversible neutralization characteristic of weak acids and bases.[16]

Just because we have pictured Ehrlich arguing an organic-chemical approach against Bordet and Arrhenius, it must not be forgotten that he was still, at heart, an experimental *biologist*. This is important, in that it helps to explain another difference between Ehrlich and Arrhenius. Arrhenius represents the "pure" or "hard" sciences of physics and chemistry, which deal with unchanging laws of nature and adhere closely to the parsimony of Occam's razor. But, as Ernst Mayr has pointed out,[17] biology demands a different philosophical approach from that of chemistry or physics; the molecules of chemistry and the particles of physics have no evolutionary history like the molecules of biology. Moreover, evolution has added layer upon layer of mechanistic complexity, of alternate pathways, and of feedback controls onto most biological processes. This may help to explain why Paul Ehrlich would feel free to argue for a highly complex set of components and interactions in this most biological of systems, the interaction of toxin with antitoxin.

THE INITIAL FORMULATION: TOXINS
AND TOXOIDS

The initial observation that posed a conceptual problem to Ehrlich was the discrepancy between the values of L_0 and L_+,[18] as we saw in the last chapter. It will be recalled that Ehrlich defined one "immunity unit" of antitoxin as that amount that would just neutralize 100 lethal doses of diphtheria toxin.[19] In assaying toxin solutions, he chose two endpoints: L_0, the amount of toxin solution just neutralized by one unit of antiserum and L_+, the amount of toxin solution that, when added to one unit of antiserum, would leave one lethal dose free to kill the experimental animal. Obviously, $L_+ - L_0$ should equal one lethal dose—but it almost never did; it usually yielded values appreciably greater than one. In addition, the value of $L_+ - L_0$ in a given solution of toxin was not constant, but would often increase over time.

How could this be explained? It rapidly became apparent to Ehrlich that the toxin was unstable, changing into a nontoxic product that he named *toxoid*. But whereas the toxicity of the preparation appeared to diminish with time, its ability to react with the antiserum remained more-or-less intact—that is, the toxoid maintains its ability to combine with antibody. This implied to Ehrlich that the portion of the toxin molecule that binds to antibody (Ehrlich's postulated receptor on sensitive cells) and the portion of the molecule responsible for toxicity are different. He named the former the *haptophore group* and the latter the *toxophore group*. Here was the chemist once again, who pictured both antigens and antibodies as complex molecules with different functional side-groups responsible for different biological/chemical functions. His later pictures of these molecules (see Chapter 6) would always show the attachment sites for antigen and complement in different parts of the antibody molecule, and the attachment sites of complement or toxin as different from their active hemolytic or toxic sites.

It was immediately clear to Ehrlich that all solutions of diphtheria toxin were in fact mixtures of variable quantities of toxin and its breakdown product, toxoid. But in his discussion of the conditions under which the molecule loses its toxicity and becomes toxoid, Ehrlich suggests that combining (haptophore) groups with different affinities[20] for the antibody may be formed. He can conceive of three types: one with greater affinity than the original toxin, which he names *protoxoid;* one with an equal affinity *(syntoxoid);* and one with a lower affinity *(epitoxoid).* By analogy with the neutralization of mixtures of hydrochloric and acetic acids by sodium hydroxide, he suggests that the neutralization of toxin-toxoid mixtures by antibody follows similar rules. The high affinity molecules are neutralized first, and then those of lower affinity. Ehrlich then gives examples of how the addition of toxin preparations containing different proportions of the several postulated toxoids may affect the value of $L_0 - L_+$.[21]

Ever on the lookout for mathematical precision, Ehrlich now attempts to quantify the analysis of toxin preparations. He claims that it is the presence of low-affinity epitoxoids that affect the value of $L_0 - L_+$, and thus the composition of any toxin preparation may be represented by x[pro- + syn-toxoids] + y[toxin] + z[epitoxoid].

Apparently casting about to rationalize the varying values of $L_0 - L_+$ that he has found experimentally, he makes two *ad hoc* assumptions: first, that epitoxoids are formed *de novo* and not from the breakdown of toxin; and, second, that toxin is transformed into protoxoid and syntoxoid, but only in a ratio of either 1:1 or 2:1! Utilizing these assumptions and numbers, Ehrlich reanalyzes his experimental results and concludes that the 'unit' of antitoxin can actually neutralize 200 lethal doses of toxin rather than the 100 doses originally postulated, the difference being due to the invariable presence in these mixtures of some 100 units of the several toxoids.

Here was the start of what became, in Ehrlich's hands, an ever-increasingly complex explanation of the mechanism of interaction of diphtheria toxins and toxoids with their specific antibody. The complexity of Ehrlich's interpretation of the neutralization of toxin mixtures by antitoxin increased significantly in his next publication on the subject, in 1899.[22] First, he gave the new name "toxon" to "epitoxoid," to emphasize that it is an original product of the bacillus and not a secondary breakdown product of toxin; it possesses, in addition, an intrinsic mild toxicity. Next, he finds it necessary to explain how a given toxin can break down into two different toxoids (pro- and syn-toxoids) of differing avidities.[23] To this end, he feels constrained to postulate that toxins may also have different avidities; he speaks, in order of decreasing avidity, of prototoxins, deuterotoxins, and tritotoxins (and of their respective toxoids), and of α and β modifications of these toxins, depending on whether they are more or less stable. Finally, he introduces the terms *hemitoxin* for those toxins that have decomposed by some 50% to toxoids, and *mesotoxin* for those toxins that have undergone no decomposition to toxoid.

Ehrlich is now ready to introduce his graphic ("mathematical") representation of the steps in the neutralization of toxin mixtures by antitoxin. These he calls a *Giftspektrum*, or "poison spectrum," by which he will describe the stepwise neutralization by antibody of the multiple components of the toxin mixture, remembering that the mixture representing the L_0 dose always contains 200 neutralizing units of haptophore combining groups. Typical examples of these graphical representations are illustrated in Figure 5.1.

Several aspects of Ehrlich's concept become clear from a consideration of these neutralization sequences. He views the toxin preparation as a mixture of discrete molecular entities, some toxic and others not, but all possessing a haptophore group able to interact with antibody. Further, following his early view of the firm (organic-chemical) binding of substance with receptor, he assumes that each substance of higher affinity will be completely bound to antibody before initiation of the neutralization of those components of lesser affinity. Finally, in view of this latter assumption, the neutralization takes the form, not of a continuous curve, but of a discontinuous bar diagram.

Here was Ehrlich introducing a congeries of hypothetical substances to support his ambition to put diphtheria assays on a firm mathematical basis. It was quite clear that toxoid exists, representing a molecule that has lost its toxic properties while retaining its ability to interact with antitoxic antibody. But the existence of the postulated toxins and toxoids of different combining affinities, and of

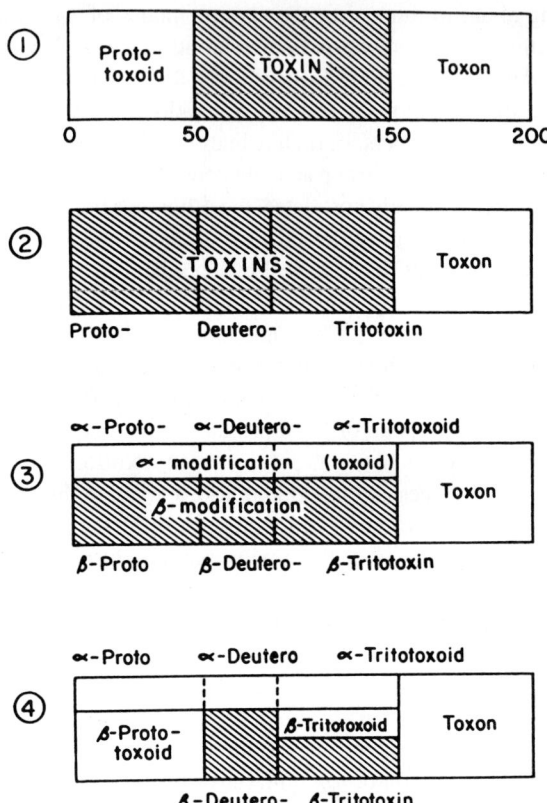

FIGURE 5.1   Ehrlich's "Giftspectrum" for the neutralization of diphtheria toxin by antitoxin. With time, the toxin is modified into the several components of different affinities. The toxins occupy the shaded areas, the nontoxic products the unshaded areas. (After Aschoff, L., *Ehrlichs Seitenkettentheorie und ihre Anwendung auf die Künstlichen Immunisierungsprozesse,* Jena, Gustav Fischer, 1902.)

the rule of toxin breakdown in the proportions of one-half or two-thirds is nowhere experimentally demonstrated; they are pragmatically chosen to provide a "best fit" to the data and lend to the method the air of mathematical certainty. Fortunately, the practical value of Ehrlich's protocol for the standardization of diphtheria toxins and antitoxins did not depend on the validity of his theoretical concepts. But the many components of Ehrlich's "poison spectrum," and even the form of the graphs themselves, were sure to pique the curiosity of, and to raise objections from, other scientists; this was not long in coming.

THE EHRLICH–BORDET DEBATE

We have seen that Ehrlich's view of the antigen–antibody interaction was based on the idea that its specificity depends on the tight chemical joining of two complementary structures. As Ehrlich would say, using the famous simile of Emil Fischer, they "fit" one another like lock and key (but there are no master keys in this system, as Pauline Mazumdar has made clear).[24] Jules Bordet, however, found fault with Ehrlich's formulation on three main grounds:

1. On the operational level, Bordet objected to the large number of different substances postulated by Ehrlich. He argued for a more Ockhamian simplicity, as Arrhenius also would.
2. On the epistemological level, Bordet criticized Ehrlich's "audacious synthetic concepts"; Bordet's ideas, he claims, are not theories, but "merely represent a description of the true state of affairs."[25]
3. On the semantic level, Bordet would criticize Ehrlich's nomenclature, claiming that the terms he employed (such as *Amboceptor, Zwischenkörper,* and *Komplement* implied too much about mechanism. Bordet preferred the more neutral terms *anticorps* and *alexine,* and would refer to hemolytic anti-erythrocyte antibody as the *substance sensibilisatrice.*[26]

That it should have been Bordet from within the immunological community who disputed Ehrlich on the mechansms of humoral immunity is an irony that has not escaped historians.[27] The young Bordet had come from Belgium to learn immunology in the laboratory of Elie Metchnikoff, whose cellular immunology fiercely opposed Ehrlich and the humoralists. It was from this hotbed of cellularism at the Pasteur Institute that Bordet reported on one of the most significant contributions to humoralist theory, the demonstration of antibody-mediated hemolysis.[28]

Bordet could not accept Ehrlich's chemical interpretation of antibody–antigen binding as involving the interaction of stereochemically complementary structures. He preferred a more physical adsorptive process, analogous to the way that dyes adhere to their substrates. In this respect, Bordet followed the lead of Karl Landsteiner in viewing the process as a colloidal reaction,[29] and would later explain the Danysz effect[30] by comparison with the stepwise adsorption of the dye methyl violet onto filter paper.[31] When it was suggested that adsorptive colloidal processes could not account for the fine specificity of immunological reactions, Bordet countered, "The affinity of adsorption is sufficiently delicate, graduated, and elective, so that the notion of its participation in antigen-antibody reactions is compatible with that of specificity."[32]

Perhaps the greatest difference between Bordet and Ehrlich lay in their scientific styles (it was surely not in the quality of their contributions to immunology, for both would be recognized with Nobel Prizes, Ehrlich in 1908 and Bordet in 1919). Ehrlich had a theory to explain every observation, whereas Bordet pretended that any ideas that he might have advanced were not even worthy to be called theories, but "merely represent a description of the true state of affairs." He would write,

> one knows with what luxuriance they [theories] have been developed on the fertile ground of immunology, where so much of the unknown still stimulates the imagination and invites audaciously synthetic concepts from the schools desirous of affirming their superiority ... conceptions that are defended with all of the partisanship that *amour propre* mixed with chauvinism so readily inspires.[33]

Despite their differences, each of the protagonists held the other in high regard and they were never reduced to unseemly polemic and *ad hominem* accusations. Each credited the other with having helped to stimulate progress in this increasingly important discipline.

THE EHRLICH–ARRHENIUS DEBATE

Thorvald Madsen earned his M.D. degree from the University of Copenhagen in 1893, and became an assistant to the noted bacteriologist Carl Julius Salomonsen. He worked on the difficult problem of the standardization of diphtheria antitoxic serum and in 1896 wrote his doctoral dissertation on this subject.[34] The work attracted the attention of Ehrlich, who cited Madsen in his landmark paper on the standardization of serotherapeutic reagents.[35] Thenceforth, Madsen made many working visits to Ehrlich's institute, and the two developed a mutual friendship and admiration; Madsen was one of the few foreigners invited to contribute to the 1914 Festschrift in honor of Ehrlich's 60th birthday.[36]

In 1899, Madsen went off on the customary *Wanderjahr,* but chose (unusual for a physician already committed to bacteriology) to devote the time to learning physical chemistry. Part of the period was spent in Stockholm with the already famous Svante Arrhenius, who by then had developed a theory of electrolytic dissociation that was to win him the Nobel Prize for chemistry in 1903. Following frequent visits to Madsen in Copenhagen, Arrhenius became interested in serotherapy and in Ehrlich's interpretation of the nature of the interaction of diphtheria toxin with antitoxin.[37] With the full force and prestige of the laws of chemistry and physics behind him, Arrhenius felt sure that he could bring order into the poorly understood and theoretically immature biological sciences. As Crawford says, "he was also committed to making serotherapy and immunity studies more scientific, using the concepts and methods of physical chemistry."[38]

In 1901 and again in 1902, Arrhenius spent a month with Madsen in Copenhagen, designing and undertaking experiments and discussing the implications of their results. Madsen taught Arrhenius the technics and reagents of the system, and Arrhenius fit the data to equations and plotted them as the typical curves of the physical chemist. The results of this work were published in the celebratory volume prepared for the opening of the Danish State Serum Institute in September 1902.[39] Arrhenius felt that Ehrlich's method of titrating toxin, involving *in vivo* tests employing many mice, was not only time-consuming but inexact; as a chemist, he would much prefer a more precise *in vitro* test. He and Madsen therefore chose to use as their toxin the tetanolysin elaborated by the tetanus bacillus, and as their assay of its interaction with antitetanolysin, the *in vitro* hemolysis of erythrocytes. This choice, while logical, would cause problems when they sought to challeng Ehrlich's diphtheria toxin results with their own tetanolysin data.

Arrhenius and Madsen aimed to demonstrate that mixtures of tetanolysin and antitetanolysin follow the same laws of chemical reaction as do weak acids

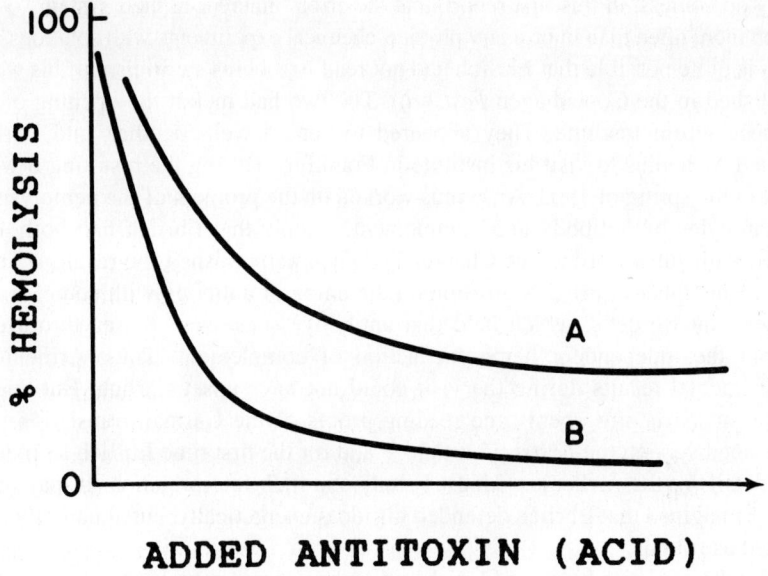

ADDED ANTITOXIN (ACID)

FIGURE 5.2   Arrhenius's comparison of the equilibrium neutralization of ammonia by boric acid (curve A) with the neutralization of tetanolysin by its specific antibody (curve B). (After Arrhenius and Madsen, note 39.)

and bases—that is, the law of mass action,[40] which implies reversibility of interaction. In line with this, they presented data suggesting that the degree of hemolysis depends on the square of lysin concentration; that the reaction velocity is proportional to the concentration of reactants; and that the influence of temperature on reaction velocity is in line with other chemical reactions and with hemolysis by alkalis. They argued that the results with tetanolysin parallel those with diphtheria toxin.

Now they are ready to attack Ehrlich's interpretation of toxin–antitoxin interactions. Why, they ask, is it necessary to plot the results in the form of Ehrlich's toxin spectrum, in which the neutralization of toxin is presented as a series of discrete steps represented by interrupted bars? Why not picture the neutralization as a continuous curve, representing a smooth *equilibrium* transition from toxic to neutral mixture, such as the physical chemist is accustomed to? They compared the curves of the neutralization of tetanolysin by its antibody to that of the neutralization of a weak acid (boric acid) by a weak base (ammonium hydroxide) (Fig. 5.2), and concluded that there was "striking agreement" between the two. This means that the toxin–antitoxin relationship should be represented by the familiar reversible equation of physical chemistry,

toxin + antitoxin ↔ toxin-antitoxin complex

They do confess, in this first report, that the errors inherent in their system "occur much more often than in ordinary physico-chemical experiments with solutions."[41]

It is quite possible that Ehrlich had not read Arrhenius's criticism of his work, published in the Copenhagen *Festskrift*. The two had met at the opening of the Danish Serum Institute. They appeared to get on well together, and Ehrlich invited Arrhenius to visit his institute in Frankfurt. During the resulting 6-week visit in the spring of 1903, Arrhenius worked on the problem of the hemolysis of erythrocytes by antibody and complement, a topic that Ehrlich had hotly disputed with Jules Bordet (see Chapter 7). When he published the results 4 years later,[42] he upheld Ehrlich's position on the union of antibody with complement, rather than Bordet's, which held that antibody "sensitizes" the erythrocyte to permit the independent hemolytic action of complement. Thus, Arrhenius's experimental results during the visit could not have upset Ehrlich. But during this visit, Arrhenius spent time reading proofs of the German translation of a shortened version the *Festskrift* article,[43] and for the first time Ehrlich learned of the details of the Arrhenius–Madsen study and their interpretation. It may readily be imagined that Ehrlich defended his ideas energetically, but apparently they parted as friends.[44]

But the armistice between Ehrlich and Arrhenius was soon broken by the intercession of one of Ehrlich's principal *bêtes noires,* Max von Gruber. Gruber had for several years been attacking Ehrlich's side-chain theory and his concept of the nature of toxin–antitoxin interactions, and Ehrlich had felt called upon to respond—somewhat contemptuously—to each published attack.[45] Then, during the summer of 1903, Gruber published a satire on Ehrlich's concept,[46] purporting to come from a "Dr. Peter Phantasus *by God's Grace Chemist,*" which included a *Giftspektrum* describing the "toxic" action of distilled water, which lyses erythrocytes due to osmotic disruption, including even the suggested formation of toxoids. However, what especially stung Ehrlich was Gruber's postscript, which announced that Arrhenius, "the famous discoverer of electrolytic dissociation" and Madsen, "a most meticulous bacteriologist" had "put the phantom of the side-chain theory to rest."

Ehrlich was quick to respond, and he replied not only to Gruber's attack, but now somewhat bitingly also to Arrhenius's implied challenge. In his reply to Gruber, Ehrlich took to task "such authors as Gruber, who have absolutely no personal experience in the main questions, [but] wage a bitter war merely because they have made a few literary studies."[47] In a frustrated response to Gruber's repeated attacks, Ehrlich would eventually declare: "In a way, therefore, my position is like that of a chess player who, even though his game is won, is forced by the obstinacy of his opponent to carry on move by move until the final 'mate.'"[48]

At the outset, Ehrlich was somewhat more circumspect in dealing with Arrhenius. He had his assistant Julius Morgenroth, a close friend of Arrhenius, write to the latter urging him to dissociate himself from Gruber's attacks and not to keep such 'bad company.' Morgenroth also suggested that Arrhenius and Madsen might even write an article against Gruber, but Arrhenius did not even answer these letters. Thus, Ehrlich felt forced to respond not only to Gruber, but to clarify once again his position vis-à-vis the criticisms of Arrhenius and Madsen.[49] He wrote a long, three-part review of his ideas, defending them in detail against the Arrhenius–Madsen attack.[50] To soften the blow however, especially with respect to Madsen, Ehrlich opened the article by congratulating Madsen for having succeeded in attracting a distinguished physical chemist to the study of toxins and antitoxins, something that Ehrlich had failed to accomplish in Germany despite years of effort.

Ehrlich first summarizes the Arrhenius–Madsen results, and then points out that he himself had earlier demonstrated also the effect of concentration and temperature on the rate of toxin neutralization. More specifically, he suggests that the tetanolysin system may not precisely parallel the diphtheria toxin sytem, since the affinity of the former is so much weaker than that of the latter. Further, he points out that in pure chemistry it is a general rule that to make precise measurements it is necessary to deal with pure substances, or at least with substances whose degree of purity is known. But these toxin preparations are not pure, nor is their exact composition known; how then, Ehrlich implies, can one treat them using the exact laws of chemistry, as Arrhenius had done?[51]

Ehrlich then proceeds to analyze in detail a large amount of data in the context of his notions about the multiplicity of toxins and toxoids, arguing in each instance that the results support his notions and contradict those of Arrhenius. He reviews the manner in which toxin decomposes into toxoid and, ever the structural chemist, engages in a fascinating discussion of the possibility that such a transformation may be accompanied by changes in avidity.[52] Ehrlich recalls that in his original publication,[53] he had assumed that there is a single species of toxin and multiple species of toxoid breakdown products. He now provides an interpretation of this phenomenon. Following up on his concept of distinct toxophore and haptophore groups on the molecule, he suggests that if these groups are widely separated, then deterioration of the toxic moiety should not affect the binding group, and thus it should leave its avidity unchanged. However, should these groups lie close together on the parent molecule, then a change in the toxophore may result in a change in the avidity of the neighboring haptophore for its antibody, either enhancing or reducing its binding ability. (Here is an interesting foretaste of the discussion 60 years later of allosteric conformational changes induced in the binding affinity of the active site on antibody or enzymes.)[54] In analyzing his newer data, however, Ehrlich concludes that the different avidities of the several toxoids originate in the breakdown of different species of toxin, each with its own avidity that remains unchanged on the daughter toxoid.

Finally, Ehrlich argues strongly for the existence of toxon, against the objections of Arrhenius and Madsen. Without his postulated toxon, Ehrlich suggests that he cannot adequately explain the neutralization spectrum of diphtheria toxin. Indeed, he reanalyzes some earlier published data of Dreyer and Madsen[55] and suggests that it can only be properly interpreted by the inclusion of toxon. At the end of the paper, Ehrlich summarizes his position as follows:

1. The diphtheria bacillus produces different types of poisons, especially toxins and toxons.
2. The avidity of diphtheria toxins for antitoxin is high.
3. The deviation of the graph of toxin neutralization from a continuous curve is not attributable to the assumption of a single toxin of weak affinity, but rather to the presence of a mixture of different toxins and toxoids.
4. The different avidities of the several toxoids is not due to changes in the avidity of a single toxin during its change to toxoid, but rather to the presence of preformed toxins of differing avidities.
5. No change in [the avidity of] the haptophore group occurs during toxoid formation.
6. The absolute number of binding units in the "immunity unit" (*Immunitätseinheit,* or L_0 dose) is 200.

Having so strongly defended his position against the attack of Arrhenius, Ehrlich adds a final paragraph to this lengthy discourse, to soften the blow. He points out that it is not surprising to encounter "a certain interference" at the outset when two such special fields meet, with their differing mathematic-physical and biological points of view. Physical chemistry must strive to employ the fewest factors possible in its computations, whereas biological analysis must deal with the "wondrous diversity" of organic substances. "I believe and hope that the unification of the two directions will be very much possible and salutory." Biology must adapt to mathematical methods and utilize only the minimal number of concepts, but the physical chemist must take into consideration that this minimal multiplicity [of assumptions] is experimentally determined. The task will be difficult, so that they must work closely together. Ehrlich closes by stating that he "takes it for a great gain that so distinguished a leader as Svante Arrhenius has taken an active interest in our area, and has associated himself in a joint undertaking with my friend and student Th. Madsen."[56]

THE DEBATE CONTINUES

After the initial salvo from both sides, the debate between Ehrlich and Arrhenius settled down primarily to a war of words. For his part, Ehrlich saw fit to publish in the *Berliner klinische Wochenschrift* the pertinent portion of a letter to Arrhenius, in which he reviewed his position and reinterpreted his data to demonstrate the validity of his conclusions.[57] Ehrlich implied to this wider readership that they can appreciate the validity of his position, even if Arrhenius cannot.

The next salvo from Ehrlich came on a trip to the United States in 1904, where he had been invited to give the Herter Lectures at the Johns Hokins University in Baltimore. This was a series of three lectures, whose summaries from notes were published in the *Boston Medical and Surgical Journal*.[58] The first lecture was entitled "The mutual relations between toxin and antitoxin," in which Ehrlich reviewed the history and essence of his side-chain theory and his concept of the nature of toxins, toxoids, and antitoxins, and their interactions. In the second lecture, entitled "Physical chemistry v. biology in the doctrines of immunity," Ehrlich outlined in detail the methods that he employs and the excellent fit to the data afforded by his many postulated toxins and toxoids—this in contrast to the questionable validity of Arrhenius's assumptions and the paucity of the data that he and Madsen presented to support them. The third lecture in this series relates to the mechanism of immune hemolysis and his debate thereon with Jules Bordet, and will be taken up in the next chapter.

The last major component of Ehrlich's polemical exchange with Arrhenius was written in collaboration with his student Hans Sachs.[59] It was an obvious effort to bring Ehrlich's views and methods to the attention of a wider chemical public. The authors point out the difference between chemical and biological analysis, in view of the complexity and impurity of biological substances. "When the doors of chemistry are provisionally closed, so can and must the biologist seek to provide clarity by means of experiment." They go on to review the highlights of Ehrlich's theory, and the arguments in support of his views of the nature of toxin–antitoxin interactions and in opposition to those of Arrhenius. They do admit, however, that there may be an initial reversibility to the interaction, but that this is soon followed by a "secondary strengthening" of the binding.[60]

Arrhenius, for his part, answered these attacks by Ehrlich with only a brief rebuttal in the literature.[61] He chose, rather, to take his position to the scientific public in a series of lectures throughout Europe and the United States. By this time, he was further armed with added prestige conferred by receipt of the 1903 Nobel Prize for chemistry. The first of these lectures took place at the German Bunsen Society meeting in Bonn in May 1904, where Arrhenius was scheduled to debate with Ehrlich in public. However, the plot was further complicated by the presence of the distinguished physical chemist Walther Nernst. Nernst had arrived (supposedly at the instigation of Ehrlich) to attack Arrhenius's position, arguing from the point of view of the increasingly popular colloid chemistry.[62] In this criticism of Arrhenius,[63] he sought to show that the data in the tetanolysin system did not support the application of the law if mass action. As Nernst said, "the concept of a reversible process collides with the facts of immunity theory."[64] In his own lecture, Arrhenius not only repeated his standard attack on Ehrlich, but attempted to undercut Nernst's argument by modifying his original equation.[65] Instead of

$$\text{antitoxin } (A) + \text{toxin } (T) \leftrightarrow AT$$

he proposed that the equation should be

$$A + T \leftrightarrow A'T' + B$$

where *B* represents a by-product of the reaction. But Nernst refused to accept this *ad hoc* modification, which he said was advanced only to preserve Arrhenius's theoretical position.

From Bonn, Arrhenius continued his immunological lectures in Holland, France, and England, and then in the United States. He found support for his position at the Pasteur Institute in Paris and at the Lister Institute in London; the support from the French may have been less pro-Arrhenius than anti-Ehrlich.[66] Then, in the summer of 1904, Arrhenius gave a lecture course on the application of physical chemistry to serum therapy at the University of California at Berkeley. The invitation was made at the suggestion of the noted biologist Jacques Loeb; other invitees for the summer session included chemist William Ramsay and geneticist Hugo de Vries. Based in part on the Berkeley lectures, Arrhenius wrote, over the next two years, a book to explain his views on the problems of immunity. He had originally thought to entitle the book *The Physical Chemistry of Antibodies,*[67] but finally ended with the felicitous new coinage, *Immunochemistry.* He hoped, as the introduction states, "to indicate ... the chemical reactions of the substances that are produced by the injection of foreign substances into the blood of animals, i.e., by immunization."[68]

Arrhenius addressed his book primarily to the medical profession, hoping to convince them of the importance of chemical thinking and chemical methodology in biological research. The presentation of his thesis was more pedagogical than polemical, and therefore his attack on Ehrlich's ideas was not especially severe. He first outlined some of the important general principles of physical chemistry, including reaction rates in homogeneous and heterogeneous systems and the nature of reversible reactions, using complement-mediated hemolysis as an example. He argued that since toxins and antitoxins diffuse like other molecules, they should be subject to van't Hoff's law of osmotic pressure and therefore to Guldberg and Waage's law of mass action. With little actual data to support the idea, he implied that those who opposed it bore the onus of disproving it. In the absence of such refutation, he felt justified in saying that, "it seems to me very unphilosophical *a priori* to suppose that other laws should regulate the reaction of toxins and antitoxins than those which govern the reactions of other substances."[69]

Arrhenius then discussed immune hemolysis in detail, touching on the debate between Ehrlich and Bordet over mechanism. In brief, he sided with Bordet in questioning the complexity of Ehrlich's theories of the antigen-complement-erythrocyte interaction (or of the toxin–antitoxin interaction), but had to agree with Ehrlich in questioning Bordet's claim that colloidal adsorption processes dominate the phenomenon.

In the years that followed publication of *Immunochemistry,* the fine points of the Ehrlich-Arrhenius debate were not often mentioned prominently in the journals. Only in the 1914 Festschrift dedicated to Ehrlich did his assistant Hans Aronson revisit minutely the Ehrlich notions and the Arrhenius challenge, concluding (understandably) that Ehrlich was correct in all particulars.[70] For his part Madsen, in a chapter in the same volume on quantitative methods in toxin research, omitted completely the battle over theoretical interpretations.[71] Interestingly, Marx reviewed the recent literature on toxins in the same volume,[72] and concluded that while the interaction of toxin and antitoxin is reversible *in the initial stages,* the binding later becomes irreversible![73] This was based in part on the demonstration by Martin and Cherry[74] that free toxin could be separated from neutral mixtures by filtration through gelatin for the first few hours after addition of antitoxin, and not thereafter. However, he called attention to Morgenroth's demonstration that cobratoxin could be isolated from neutral mixtures for a long time, using hydrochloric acid to split the antigen–antibody complex.[75] Marx then discussed the "paradoxical" activity of antitoxins in the so-called Danysz phenomenon,[76] in which the stepwise addition of antitoxin to a toxin solution leads to a lesser degree of neutralization than does addition all at once. This observation would also appear to argue against Arrhenius's suggestion that the toxin–antitoxin interaction is simple and reversible.

In the final analysis, Arrhenius's book *Immunochemistry* exerted little influence on contemporary immunological research. Perhaps the times were not yet ready for the application of the "hard" sciences to this area of biomedicine; while a few chemical journals reviewed the book (its author was, after all, a Nobel Prize winner for chemistry), few biological or medical journals mentioned it, and few researchers in immunity followed Arrhenius's suggestions. Thus, its principal contribution was the introduction of the term "immunochemistry," and only some half-century later would Arrhenius's ambition to apply rigorous chemistry to immunological problems be realized, in the hands of Landsteiner, Heidelberger, Pauling, Karush, and others.

NOBEL PRIZE IMPLICATIONS
OF THE DISPUTE

The dispute over toxins and antitoxins was not restricted to the podia at scientific meeting or to the pages of the pertinent journals. It also entered the halls of the Karolinska Institute in Stockholm, where the Nobel Prize committees considered candidates for the various prizes that were conferred starting in 1901. Svante Arrhenius figured significantly over many years in the evaluation of candidates for the prize in Physiology or Medicine, and Ehrlich's candidacy would suffer from Arrhenius's opposition. This story, which reflects little credit on Arrhenius, is told by Crawford in her biography *Arrhenius*[77] and in even greater detail in Franz Luttenberger's study of the Ehrlich/Arrhenius controversy and its implications for the Nobel Prize.[78] In brief, Arrhenius, as one of the founders of physical chemistry, as a 1903 Nobel Prize winner himself, and as one of the leaders of Stockholm science, was able to exert appreciable influence on the considerations of the committee responsible for evaluating and recommending candidates, even though not himself a committee member. He did this in part through his own prestigious influence, and in part through his brother-in-law, physiologist Johan Erik Johansson, who was then chairman of the medical Nobel Committee.

Ehrlich was first nominated for the Nobel Prize in 1901, when it was awarded to Behring. He was seriously considered starting in 1902, and increasingly thereafter. Over the years, Ehrlich received a total 70 nominations from 13 countries, but each year his nomination failed because of the questions raised by Arrhenius's objections to Ehrlich's theories. When, in time, consideration of Ehrlich for the prize in medicine became stronger, Johansson delivered renewed attacks on the Ehrlich candidacy, apparently written by Arrhenius. Finally, however, and due in part to the support that Ehrlich received from Walther Nernst, which helped to neutralize the Arrhenius position, the Prize for 1908 was awarded to Ehrlich, but only to be shared with Elie Metchnikoff.

Starting in 1913, Ehrlich was once again nominated for the prize, this time for his chemotherapeutic studies and for Salvarsan. However, Ehrlich's death in 1915 rendered this issue moot. In his description of the Nobel Prizes in physiology or medicine, Göran Liljestrand[79] seems to imply that Ehrlich might well have received a second Nobel Prize, had he lived long enough. One wonders whether, had Ehrlich lived, Arrhenius would have fought this second nomination too.

Arrhenius was not done, however. Just as he had disagreed with Ehrlich, so he had serious disagreement with Nernst, whose championing of colloidal interpretations appeared to threaten Arrhenius's contributions to physical chemistry. In addition, Nernst had challenged Arrhenius directly by defending Ehrlich. Thus, when Nernst's name came up for serious consideration as early as 1909, Arrhenius fought it then and for many years thereafter, and repeatedly wrote reports to the committee questioning the value of Nernst's work. But eventually Arrhenius's influence waned, and Nernst's important contributions to thermochemistry were recognized by award of the Nobel Prize for chemistry in 1920 (awarded in 1921).

The history of the Nobel candidacies of Ehrlich and Nernst referred to, and that of Elie Metchnikoff as outlined by Tauber in his review of Nobel archives,[80] demonstrate how politicized the awards might be. They show also how personalities, differences in scientific style, and even questions of nationalism may influence the process.

THE FINAL RESOLUTION OF THEORY
AND PRACTICE

The modern history of toxin–antitoxin research confirms yet again one of the truisms of the biomedical sciences; in most serious disputes, both sides will usually prove to have been partially correct in their views. Thus, Ehrlich was ultimately shown to be correct in his claim that according to the side-chain theory, the toxin molecule possesses two separate stereochemical groups, the toxophore and haptophore, and that the former could be "detoxified" to form toxoid without disturbing the binding capacity of the molecule. Ehrlich was also partially correct in suggesting that the neutralization of toxin by antitoxin involves molecules of varying combining affinity, but whereas he attributed this heterogeneity to different toxin and toxoid species, it would later be shown that it was the antibody that was heterogeneous.[81] This would prove to depend on the activation of many different clones of antibody-forming B cells following immunization by a single antigenic epitope.[82]

But Ehrlich was wrong and Arrhenius right on the question of the reversibility of the antigen–antibody bond. Ehrlich had thought that the bond was firm like the carbon-carbon bond of organic chemistry, because once formed, the antigen–antibody complex seemed almost immutable. The reason for this became clear, when J.R. Marrack proposed that antibodies are divalent and form a tight lattice wherein the complex multiple attachments firmly anchor the molecules in place.[83] The case for the reversibility of the interaction of a *single* antibody combining site with its antigenic epitope developed initially with the demonstration of hapten inhibition of precipitin formation and then with the demonstration by Pauling and Pressman of the nature of the antigen–antibody bond, composed of contributions by electrostatic, hydrogen bonding, and van der Waals interactions.[84]

As to the practical medical aspects of diphtheria and tetanus antitoxin serotherapy, this approach continued to save many lives with complete disregard for the theoretical disputes previously described. Ehrlich's recipe for toxin–antitoxin standardization, or some modification of it, continued to serve the therapeutic community. However, in 1906, Clemens von Pirquet and Bela Schick made it clear that the administration of horse antitoxin (or other xenogeneic product) was not without danger.[85] They described the development in serotherapy patients of *serum sickness,* a disease involving glomerulonephritis and other systemic problems, due to the formation of immune complexes that follow the host's immune response to horse serum proteins. At the same time, improvements were made in the quality of toxoid preparations and in vehicles (alum precipitation, etc.) for the enhancement of immunogenicity,[86] so that the prophylactic induction of *active* immunity became a much-preferred option. With the introduction of obligatory childhood DPT immunization (against diphtheria, pertussis, and tetanus), the use of passive serotherapy has substantially disappeared, except for the use of human immune globulin in preventing maternal Rh sensitization and erythroblastosis fetalis, or in the treatment of such diseases as infectious hepatitis.

NOTES AND REFERENCES

1. Pasteur, L., C. Chamberland, and E. Roux, *C.R. Acad. Sci.* 90:239, 1880.
2. Grawetz, P., *Virchows Archiv.* 84:87, 1881. See also Behring, E. *Deutsch. med. Wochenschr.* 16:1145, 1890.
3. Behring, E. and Kitasato, S., *Deutsch. med. Wochenschr.* 16:1113, 1890.
4. Buchner, H., *Münch. med. Wochenschr.* 40:449, 480, 1893; Roux, E. and Vaillard, L., *Ann. Inst. Pasteur* 7:65, 1894.
5. Ehrlich showed that ricin could agglutinate erythrocytes (*Fortschr. Med.* 15:41, 1897), and that they could be hemolyzed by tetanolysin (*Berlin. klin. Wochenschr.* 35:273, 1898). Bordet also demonstrated agglutination and hemolysis with anti-erythrocyte antibodies (*Ann. Inst. Pasteur* 12:688, 1898).
6. Morgenroth, J., *Berlin klin. Wochenschr.* 42:1550, 1905.

7. This situation had actually arisen once before. In the debate over the mechanism of acquired immunity, Metchnikoff would employ certain pathogens and experimental approaches that favored his cellular (phagocytic) concept, while investigators in Koch's laboratory would use other approaches and pathogens more susceptible to the action of humoral antibodies. The dispute is discussed in detail in Silverstein, A.M., *Cell. Immunol.* 48:208, 1979.

8. See, for example, Fruton, J., *Contrasts in Scientific Style; Research Groups in the Chemical and Biochemical Sciences,* Philadelphia, American Historical Society, 1990, and Fruton's earlier study of styles in scientific speculation, "The emergence of biochemistry," *Science* 192:327–334, 1976; also J. Harwood, *Styles of Scientific Thought: The German Genetic Community. 1900–1933.* Chicago, University of Chicago Press, 1993; a bibliography on the subject may be found on pp. 9–17 of Harwood's book.

9. Ludwik Fleck long ago pointed out that *within* a discipline, the different approaches to a problem often depend on the 'thought-style' promulgated by the leaders of the group to which one belongs (*Genesis and Development of a Scientific Fact,* Chicago, University of Chicago Press, 1979; first published in German in 1935). Thomas Kuhn took up the thesis, and pointed out that most of the time a scientist is almost a prisoner within the conceptual and technological bounds of the "normative science" that currently dominate his or her discipline (*The Structure of Scientific Revolutions,* 2nd ed., Chicago, University of Chicago Press, 1970).

10. Jerne, N.K., "Waiting for the end," *Cold Spring Harbor Symp. Quant. Biol.* 32:591, 1967.

11. The incommensurable languages employed by the two camps has been discussed in Silverstein, A.M., *Cell. Immunol.* 97:173, 1986.

12. Mayr, E. in Mayr and Provine, W.B., eds., *The Evolutionary Synthesis: Perspectives on the Unification of Biology,* Cambridge, Harvard University Press, 1980, pp. 1–48. It may be argued that recent years have seen a similar coming together of Jerne's *cis*- and *trans*-immunologists, in what we might term an "immunological synthesis."

13. Rubin, L.P., *J. Hist. Med.* 35:397, 1980.

14. Crawford, E., *Arrhenius: From the Ionic Theory to the Greenhouse Effect,* Canton, MA, Science History Publications, 1996, p. 169 ff.

15. Mazumdar, P.M.H., *Species and Specificity. An Interpretation of the History of Immunology.* New York, Cambridge University Press, 1995.

16. The later demonstration that both antigen and antibody might be multivalent would ultimately confirm that they might interact in variable proportions and form complex aggregates that *appeared* to be irreversibly joined. Only the later work with simple chemical haptens would show that the unit binding might obey the equilibrium requirements of the law of mass action.

17. Mayr, E., *Toward a New Philsophy of Biology: Observations of an evolutionist,* Cambridge, Harvard Univ. Press, 1988.

18. Ehrlich, P., *Klin. Jahrbuch,* 6:299, 1897; English transl. *Collected Papers,* vol. II, pp. 107–125. This paper also contained the first presentation of Ehrlich's side-chain theory of antibody formation and function.

19. Ehrlich adopted the measure of an "immunity unit" from Behring, whose standard toxin contained 100 lethal doses per cc; the immunity unit of antiserum was one in which 1 cc would just neutralize 1 cc of the standard toxin.

20. Ehrlich appears in what follows to employ the terms "affinity" and "avidity" indiscriminately to signify chemical binding power. Elsewhere, avidity was used in the context of the rate of toxin–antitoxin interaction and, much later, affinity would represent the thermodynamic measure of the binding of a single antibody binding site for an antigenic epitope (simple hapten), whereas avidity would represent the measure of the total interaction of multivalent antibody with a complex antigen. See Keating, P., Cambrosio, A., and McKenzie, M. on the affinity/avidity controversy in immunology in Clarke, A.E. and Fujimora, J.H., eds., *The Right Tools for the Job: At Work in Twentieth-Century Life Sciences,* Princeton, Princeton University Press, 1992, pp. 312–354.

21. Ehrlich, note 18, *Collected Papers,* vol. II, pp. 118–119.

22. Ehrlich, P., *Deutsch, med. Wochenschr.* 24:597, 1898; *Collected Papers* vol. II, pp. 126–133.

23. Note that, in this paper, Ehrlich changes his former use of affinity *(Affinität)* to avidity *(Avidität)* without explanation. See note 20.

24. Mazumdar, *Species and Specificity,* note 15 p. 205.

25. Bordet, J., *Traité de l'Immunité dans les Maladies Infectieuses,* Masson, Paris, 1920, p. vi ff. See also the summary chapter in Bordet's *Studies in Immunity* (F. Gay, transl.), New York, Wiley, 1909, pp. 496ff. The most comprehensive study of the epistemological aspects of the Ehrlich–Bordet debates is by Crist, E. and Tauber, A.I., *J. Hist. Biol.* 30:321, 1977.

26. The semantic arguments are discussed more fully in Silverstein, A.M., note 11. The language differences in connection with the mechanism of immune hemolysis will be discussed further in Chapter 7.

27. See, e.g., Tauber, A.I. and Chernyak, L., *Metchnikoff and the Origins of Immunology: From Metaphor to Theory,* Oxford, Oxford University Press, 1991; see also Bibel, D.J., *Milestones in Immunology: A Historical Exploration,* Madison, WI, Science Tech, 1988, p. 200.

28. Bordet, J., *Ann. Inst. Pasteur* 12:688, 1899.

29. See Mazumdar, note 15, p. 226. Colloids were very popular in turn-of-century Vienna (Mazumdar, p. 214 ff and Mazumdar, *Bull. Hist. Med.* 48:1, 1974). Even Hans Zinsser, in his summary of contemporary knowledge in immunology, felt called upon to invite a closing chapter on colloids to round out the discussion (*Infection and Resistance,* New York, Macmillan, 1914).

30. This was the observation that stepwise addition of antigen would neutralize antibody more efficiently than addition all at once; Danysz, J., *Ann. Inst. Pasteur* 16:331, 1902.

31. Bordet (Gay), note 25, pp. 195–196.

32. Bordet, *Traité,* note 25, p. 546.

33. Bordet, *Traité,* note 25, p. vi ff. The use of the term *chauvinism* by Bordet against German scientists in 1919 is not surprising. He had studied at the Pasteur Institute in Paris, where the French defeat in 1870 still reverberated, and had been isolated during World War I in a Belgium overrun by the Kaiser's army. A fuller description of the political undertones of the Franco-Prussian scientific dispute will be found in Silverstein, note 7.

34. Madsen, Th., *Experimentelle Untersögelser over Difterigiften,"* dissertation, University of Copenhagen, 1896.

35. Ehrlich, P., *Klin. Jahrbuch,* 6:299, 1897; English transl. *Collected Papers,* vol. II, pp. 107–125.

36. Apolant, H. ed., *Paul Ehrlich: Eine Darstellung seines wissenschaftlichen Wirkens,* Jena, Gustav Fischer, 1914, hereafter referred to as *Ehrlich Festschrift.*

37. Arrhenius's move into immunology is not surprising. He was a polymath who, in his long career, became interested in what he termed "cosmic physics" (the interaction of oceans, land masses, and the atmosphere), the role of atmospheric CO_2 in glaciation (the "greenhouse" effect—this in 1892!), the physical chemistry of volcanoes, and the cause of the aurora borealis. He even initiated studies, never completed and published, on the influence of atmospheric electricity on the onset of menses! See, for example, Crawford, *Arrhenius* note 14, and "Arrhenius," *Dictionary of Scientific Biography,* 1:296–302. 1970.

38. Crawford, *Arrhenius,* note 14, p. 170.

39. Arrhenius, S. and Madsen, T., in C.J. Salomonsen, ed., *Festskrift ved Indvielsen af Statens Serum Institut,* Copenhagen, 1902. Salomonsen became the institute's first director, and Madsen succeeded him in this post.

40. It is interesting that Niels Jerne, in his doctoral thesis at the Copenhagen State Serum Institute, used the law of mass action to derive "avidity constants" for the interaction of diphtheria antitoxin with toxin (*Acta Path. Microbiol. Scand.* Suppl. 87, 1951). He was perplexed by the observation that the avidity of the antitoxin increases on subsequent booster immunizations (today's "affinity maturation").

41. Arrhenius and Madsen, *Festskrift,* note 39, p. 8.

42. Arrhenius, S., *Immunochemistry: The Application of the Principles of Physical Chemistry to the Study of the Biological Antibodies,* New York, Macmillan, 1907.

43. Arrhenius, S. and Madsen, T., *Z. Phys. Chem.* 44:7, 1903.

44. Crawford, *Arrhenius,* note 14, p. 194.

45. For a description of this debate, see Silverstein, A.M., *A History of Immunology,* New York, Academic Press, 1989, pp. 104–107.

46. Gruber, M., *Wien. klin. Wochenschr.* 16:791, 1903.

47. Ehrlich, P., *Münch. med. Wochenschr.* 50:1428, 1465, 1903; English translation in Ehrlich's *Collected Studies in Immunity,* C. Bolduan, transl., New York, Wiley, 1906, p. 525. See also Ehrlich's counter to Gruber's response, *Münch. med. Wochenschr.* 50:2295, 1903.

48. Ehrlich, *Collected Studies,* note 47, p. viii.

49. The Morgenroth–Arrhenius and Ehrlich–Arrhenius letters, and the background thereto, are discussed in detail by Crawford, *Arrhenius,* note 14, p. 195.

50. Ehrlich, P., *Berlin klin. Wochenschr.* 40:793, 825, 848, 1903; *Collected Papers* vol. II, pp. 347–367.

51. Ehrlich, *Collected Papers,* vol. II, p. 352.

52. Ehrlich, *Collected Papers,* vol. II, p. 357 ff.

53. Ehrlich, note 35.

54. See, e.g., Koshland, D., *Ann. N.Y. Acad. Sci.* 103:630, 1963; Kabat, E.A., *Structural Concepts in Immunology and Immunochemistry,* New York, Holt, Rinehart, and Winston, 1968; and Pressman, D. and Grossberg, A.L., *The Structural Basis of Antibody Specificity,* New York, Benjamin, 1968, p. 172 ff.

55. Dreyer, G. and Madsen, Th., in Salomonsen, *Festskrift,* note 39.

56. Ehrlich, *Collected Papers* vol. II, p. 367.

57. Ehrlich, P., *Berlin. klin. Wochenschr.* 41:221, 1904; *Collected Papers,* vol. II, pp. 406–409.

58. Ehrlich, P. "The Herter Lectures," *Boston Med. Surg. J.,* 50:442, 445, 448, 1904; *Collected Papers,* vol. II, pp. 410–422.

59. Ehrlich, P. and Sachs, H., *Ueber die Beziehungen zwischen Toxin und Antitoxin und die Wege ihrer Erforschung,* Leipzig, G. Fock, 1905.

60. This is an interesting concession on Ehrlich's part, since it goes against his earlier assumption of a tight (covalent) bond. It does, however, presage one of the consequences of J.R. Marrack's "lattice theory" (*The Chemistry of Antigens and Antibodies,* London, H.M. Stationery Office, 1934), in that the initial combination of multivalent antibodies and antigens into a complex lattice would consolidate with time, and thus be more difficult to dissociate.

61. Arrhenius, S., *Berlin klin. Wochenschr.* 41:216, 1904.

62. During the 1890s, and supported by physicist Ernst Mach and physical chemist Wolfgang Pauli, a distinction was made between chemical and "physical" interactions. The latter were assumed in general to involve "colloidal" substances that were "adsorbed" in variable proportions, rather than following the classical chemical law of fixed proportions. See Mazumdar, note 29. The colloidal concept had been adopted by Jules Bordet in his debate with Ehrlich on the mechanism of immune hemolysis, of which more in Chapter 7.

63. Nernst, W., *Z. Elektrochem.* 10:377, 1904.

64. Nernst, note 63, discussion, pp. 676–677.

65. Arrhenius, S., *Z. Elektrochem.* 10:661, 668, 1904.

66. Both Bordet and Metchnikoff would have welcomed the Arrhenius criticism of Ehrlich, since both had contested his views, Bordet with respect to immune hemolysis (see Chapter 7) and Metchnikoff in the context of the cellularist-humoralist controversy (see Silverstein, note 7).

67. See Crawford, *Arrhenius,* note 14, p. 220.

68. Arrhenius, *Immunochemistry,* note 42, pp. vii–viii.

69. Arrhenius, *Immunochemistry,* note 42, p. 36.

70. Aronson, H., *Ehrlich Festschrift,* note 36, pp. 166–190.

71. Madsen, Th., *Ehrlich Festschrift,* note 36, pp. 151–158.

72. Marx, E., *Ehrlich Festschrift,* note 36, pp. 233–244.

73. See notes 16 and 60.

74. Martin, C.J. and Cherry, T., *Proc. Roy. Soc. London* 63:420, 1898.

75. Morgenroth, J., *Berlin klin. Wochenschrift,* 1905.

76. Danysz, note 30.

77. Crawford, *Arrhenius,* note 14, p. 227 ff.
78. Luttenberger, F., *Theoretical Med.* 13:137, 1992.
79. Liljestrand, G., "The Prize in Physiology," in *Nobel, the Man and His Prizes,* Stockholm, Amsterdam, Elsevier, 1962, pp. 131–343; see p. 213.
80. Tauber, A.I., *Cell. Immunol.* 139:505, 1992.
81. The heterogeneity of antibodies was studied by hapten inhibition of precipitin formation by many authors, reviewed by Pressman and Grossberg *(Structural Basis)* and Kabat *(Structural Concepts),* note 54. The case was made elegantly by the studies of equilibrium dialysis of Eisen, H.N. and Karush, F. (*J. Am. Chem. Soc.* 71:363, 1949) in which the thermodynamic values of simple chemical hapten-antibody interactions could be measured, and the heterogeneity of the antibody combining sites estimated precisely.
82. Sigal, N.H. and Klinman, N.R. (*Adv. Immunol.* 26:255, 1978) in their summary of data on the B cell clonotype repertoire, showed that there might be as many as 5000 different clonotypes in the mouse specific for the dinitrophenyl or iodo-nitrobenzoyl haptens, a degeneracy confirmed by Sharon, J., Kabat, E.A., and Morrison, S.L., who showed that of 12 hybridomas to $\alpha 1 \rightarrow 6$ dextran, no two were identical with respect to idiotype, binding affinity, or region of the epitope involved (*Molec. Immunol.* 19:375, 389, 1982). See also D.W. Talmage's suggestion of the polyclonal basis for the large repertoire of immunological specificities (*Science* 149:1643, 1959).
83. See Marrack, *The Chemistry,* note 60.
84. For references to these many studies, see Pressman and Grossberg, *Structural Basis,* note 54.
85. von Pirquet, C. and Schick, B., *Die Serumkrankheit,* Vienna, Deuticke, 1906; von Pirquet, C., *Allergy,* Chicago, American Medical Association, 1911; see also Silverstein, A.M., *Nature Immunol.* 1:453, 2000.
86. See, e.g., Ramon, G., *C.R. Soc. Biol.* 89:2, 1923; Ramon, *C.R. Soc. Biol.* 177:1338, 1923; Glenny A.T., *J. Hygiene* 24:301, 1925; Glenny and Okell, C.C., *J. Path. Bact.* 27:187, 1924; Glenny and Barr, M., *J. Path. Bact.* 34:131, 1931; 35:91, 1932.

6

THE SIDE-CHAIN
THEORY OF ANTIBODY
FORMATION

MINISTER ALTHOFF   *If you do all the work, what does Herr*
Professor Ehrlich do?

ASSISTANT   *He thinks!*

John Huston et al., filmscript,
Dr. Ehrlich's Magic Bullet, 1940

EARLY SPECULATIONS ON IMMUNOLOGY

The ability to develop resistance to further infection after an initial exposure to a disease (acquired immunity) was recognized some 2500 years ago, when Thucidides described it in connection with the plague of Athens. As he put it, "those who had recovered from the disease ... now had no fear for themselves; for the same man was never attacked twice—never at least fatally."[1] The reason for this protection was unknown, but with the rise of Christian religiosity, disease was understood to be a punishment inflicted by God for sin. In this view, those who remained healthy during an epidemic (natural immunity) could be presumed to be without sin; those who became ill and recovered to exhibit acquired immunity could be presumed to have been cleansed of their sins and did not merit further punishment when the plague returned. Disease might thus be viewed as an expiation.

A more mechanistic view of immunity arose in the Middle Ages, especially in the world of Islamic medicine. This was based on the ancient Greek view of disease as an imbalance of the humors. In the 9th century, the physician Rhazes (who had first differentiated measles from smallpox) suggested that the well-recognized lasting immunity following recovery from smallpox could be readily explained. Smallpox, he claimed, resulted from the fermentation of a supposed excess of moisture in the blood. When this moisture is driven off through the skin

---

pustules, the individual is not only cured, but no longer has the excess moisture that might support another infection![2] An analogous explanation was proposed by the Italian Girolamo Fracastoro in 1546. In his case, it was the putative contaminant of traces of menstrual blood with which we are all born that is expelled via the smallpox pustules; this being depleted in the first attack, nothing further could be expected, since the substrate for the disease was thenceforth lacking.[3] It is interesting that both Rhazes and Fracastoro, as well as their contemporaries, viewed smallpox as a benign childhood disease, in contrast to the deadly form that it appeared to acquire from the early 17th century onward.[4]

This was not the last of the interesting theories of the basis for acquired immunity, most of which depended on changing concepts of disease pathogenesis. There was a physical theory, which held that pock formation in smallpox was due to the ebulition of matter through the pores of the skin. The force of this movement was so great that it would distend the pores; forever after they would be open, so that even if further "infection" took place, there would be no consequent clinical signs (pocks), and thus no disease.[5] Another theory held that we are all at birth endowed with the seeds of every disease possible. When the seeds of a given disease are "fertilized," illness ensues, but cannot recur because the seeds for that disease have been depleted.[6] Here is an interesting early demonstration of disease specificity.

The notion that immunity depends on the depletion of some element essential to the disease process took many forms. One of the more practical emerged from Louis Pasteur's original experimental demonstration of acquired immunity in 1880. It will be recalled that, at the time, immunity was only known to follow infection or immunization with *live* pathogens. Citing the well-known cessation of bacterial growth in culture following an initial growth phase, Pasteur suggested that this was due to the exhaustion of some trace nutrients peculiar to that organism and essential to its growth. Thus, after active infection or immunization with an attenuated strain, those critical nutrients would be absent in the host, and new infection and growth of the organism a second time could not be supported. Recurrence of disease would thus be impossible.[7] This theory could not survive the later demonstration that immunity might be induced by nonreproducing toxins and toxiods.

In 1884, zoologist Ilya Metchnikoff proposed a new theory of immunity based on Darwinian evolutionary principles.[8] He suggested that those cells responsible for the digestion of foodstuffs in invertebrates had evolved into the mobile phagocytes of vertebrates, able to ingest and digest invading pathogens. These, then, were the principle actors in natural immunity and in acquired immunity as well. The theory found favor in France, where Metchnikoff was invited by Pasteur to work in his new institute in Paris, but the concept was strongly contested, especially in Germany.[9] The opposition to the cellular theory was strongly reinforced by the discovery of the antibacterial substance alexine (later named complement) in the blood,[10] and especially by the finding by Behring and Kitasato in 1890 that immunity could be transferred passively by some kind of "anti-body" present in the serum of immunized animals.[11]

While the cellularist/humoralist debate continued apace, those who believed in the importance of circulating antibodies speculated on their origin. Buchner had proposed that antibodies are altered antigen,[12] but it was soon shown that antibody formation persists in the apparent absence of antigen,[13] and that small amounts of injected antigen may give rise to much greater amounts of antibody.[14] It seemed obvious that these antibodies must be formed within and by the immunized host, but why and how? It was clear that a serious conceptual vacuum existed in the growing field of immunity research, nowhere more apparent than in the many German laboratories engaged in research on these new antibodies.

EHRLICH'S BIOLOGICAL THEORY OF SIDE CHAINS

We must, at the outset, separate completely Ehrlich's notion of how antibodies interact with their respective antigens from his concept of where and how these antibodies originate. The former, involving debates with Bordet and with Arrhenius on purely physicochemical mechanisms of interaction, is discussed in detail in the previous chapter on toxins and antitoxins, and will be touched on also in the following chapter on the mechanism of action of hemolytic antibody and complement. We are concerned here only with the origin and details of Ehrlich's side-chain theory of antibody formation.

We saw in Chapter 1 that from the very beginning of his scientific career, Ehrlich conceived of the interaction of cells with dyes, drugs, and even nutrient molecules as mediated by specific receptors.[15] These receptors occupy the position of "side chains" attached to the surface of the cell. As he (who loved Latin aphorisms) put it, *Corpora non agunt nisi fixata,* or substances do not [inter]act unless fixed. But Ehrlich went further; he pictured the interaction as a chemical process involving stereochemical structures ("specific groups of atoms") that fit together as "lock and key" in tight combination. That the reaction is purely chemical is apparent from Ehrlich's statement that "I have been able to demonstrate by test tube experiments ... that *the interaction of toxin and antibody is much more rapid in concentrated than in dilute solutions,* and also that *heat accelerates the action and cold retards it*" [his italics].[16]

Having discarded the view that antibodies derive from exogenous substances (the injected antigen), it follows therefore that they must be products of the living organism. Moreover, "the living organism can perform this task easily, often within the course of a few days, and with a multiplicity of toxins." Now Ehrlich, the modern experimental scientist, rejects any interpretation of the phenomenon of antibody formation that smacks of an outmoded mystical vitalism or even Lamarckian mechanism. Thus,

> To attribute what could be called inventive activity to the body or to its cells, enabling them to produce new groups of atoms as required, would involve a return to the concepts current in the days of [an obsolete] *Naturphilosophie.* Our knowledge of cell function and

especially of synthetic processes would lead us rather to assume that in the formation of antibodies, we are dealing with the enhancement of a normal cell function, and not with the creation at need of new groups of atoms. Physiological analogues of the group of specifically combining antibodies must exist beforehand in the organism or in its cells.[17]

Here is the epitome of modern Darwinian thinking, although Ehrlich never explicitly mentions Darwin. He cannot, of course, explain *why* receptors for toxins (i.e., specific side chains attached to the cell) have evolved, but they form for him part of a larger physiological picture. He points out, in support of this thesis, that tetanus toxin preferentially localizes in the central nervous system rather than in other visceral organs. This can only be due to the presence in the receptive tissues of specific receptors that preexist there to mediate not only the localization but also the physiological activity of the toxin. Similarly, all substances required for cell nutrition will attach to the cell and be utilized by it, by virtue of their own specific receptors. But there is a reverse side to this coin, of great theoretical interest. If the receptor for a given toxin (e.g., pathogen) is absent, notes Ehrlich, then the toxic action of that substance cannot be exerted—this may explain many instances of natural immunity!

How do we go from the existence of antigen-specific receptors on the cell surface to the presence in the immunized host of large quantities of circulating antibody? For Ehrlich, the solution is obvious; injected antigen will combine with its receptor on the cell, neutralizing the receptor and rendering it unavailable for further physiological function. However, the deficiency of this type of receptor is made good by the new formation of identical groups by the cell, "according to the well-established principle of pathology" propounded especially by Ehrlich's cousin, Carl Weigert—that of compensatory hyperplasia.[18] When further injections of antigen are made, they neutralize the newly formed receptors and further regeneration of the side chains occurs, until the excess spills over into the bloodstream in ever-increasing amounts as specific circulating antibody. This is not only compensation, but overcompensation.

Here is the first *selective* theory of antibody formation that would inspire a generation of researchers in many fields, and a series of polemical debates about its possible validity. For Ehrlich at the time, it probably did not appear to be anything special; it was merely a repeat in a new context of the same idea that he had discussed so often before in his histological studies, in his work on cell metabolism, and in his studies of the pharmacological action of alkaloids and other agents. In an 18-page publication devoted to the standardization of toxins, toxoids, and antitoxins, he inserted in the middle only two pages to explain this new elaboration of an old idea.

FURTHER DEVELOPMENT
OF THE SIDE-CHAIN THEORY

It is interesting that two years would pass during which Ehrlich made no mention of the side-chain theory, while he elaborated at length on the complex composition of diphtheria toxin and the mechanisms of its interaction with anti-toxin.[19] However, a number of observations in the literature caused Ehrlich to revisit his theory during his dedicatory address on the opening of his new Royal Institute for Experimental Therapeutics in Frankfurt.[20] It had been shown during the preceding years that antibody formation could be induced not only against a limited number of toxins, but against a variety of simple proteins, enzymes, and other innocuous substances. But even more perplexing was the finding that destructive antibodies could be formed against erythrocytes.[21] Here was an implicit challenge to the theory that receptors for all these substances prexist within the host.

Ehrlich defended his theory by first reviewing the increasingly convincing data showing that antibody could not be some sort of derivative of antigen. A single injection of a toxin might result in the formation of enough antibody to neutralize 100,000 equivalents of toxin. In addition, active immunization confers long-lasting immunity, whereas passive transfer of immune serum confers only a transient protection. Thus, it is clear that antibody must be formed within and by the host. Then Ehrlich raises two questions that will perplex immunologists for the next three-quarters of a century. The questions are posed, but not satisfactorily answered.

The first question concerns the ability to mount an immune response against complex molecules (proteins, the secretion products of bacteria, and cells) but not against crystalline alkaloids and other small molecules. If the side chains that are to become antibodies really mediate physiological functions analogous to nutrition, why then should there not be side chains for the physiologically active alkaloids as there are for plant and bacterial toxins and other proteins? Ehrlich does not address this paradox. The second difficulty posed by these data is much deeper, and will provide the basis for the dispute described later that will ultimately call the entire selectionist theory into question. If side chains are normal constituents of the cell designed to mediate physiological functions, it is understandable that there should be specific side chains for the variety of nutrients, for drugs, and perhaps even for certain enzymes and toxins. But from where do the side chains specific for egg albumin, foreign erythrocytes, or spermatozoa come? Ehrlich does not address this paradox. Toward the end of his speech, Ehrlich for the first time defines several terms that are still employed in modern immunology. He points out that if a single pure substance is used for immunization, then only a single antibody will result and one may speak of a *monovalent* antiserum. Utilizing a complex agent such as bacteria, blood cells, or a mixture of antigens will result in the formation of a *multivalent* antiserum.

Then, in 1900, came Ehrlich's most extensive elaboration of his side-chain theory. He was invited by the Royal Society of London to give the Croonian Lecture, and he used this opportunity to explain and extend his theory before a new and important public.[22] In addition, he presented for the first time a representation of his ideas in a pictorial form that would convince a generation of investigators that they could actually "see" the antibody molecule in form and function. It is significant that, after paying his respects to Jenner for the smallpox vaccine, to

Pasteur and Koch for their experimental systems, and to Behring for antitoxic antibodies, Ehrlich opens his lecture with a quote from the English physicist Clerk Maxwell. This savant had said that if he were required to symbolize the learning of our time, he would choose a meter measure, a clock, and a kilogram weight—symbols of the quantitative approach to science that he, Ehrlich, has introduced into immunity research.

Ehrlich then reviews the extensive literature that supports the view that antibodies are side chains normally present on the cells of the host that serve to mediate the physiological functions of the antigens for which they are specific. However, he now asks the critical question about the significance of these "toxophile" groups (antitoxin side chains) in the organs of the host. As he says,

> That these are in function specially designed to seize on toxins cannot be for one moment entertained. It would not be reasonable to suppose that there were present in the organism many hundreds of atom groups destined to unite with toxins, when the latter appeared, but in function really playing no part in the processes of normal life, and only arbitrarily brought into relation with them by the will of the investigator. It would indeed be highly superfluous, for example, for all our native animals to possess in their tissues atom groups deliberately adapted to unite with abrin, ricin, and crotin, substances coming from the far distant tropics.[23]

This same question would be raised for the next 60 years, first by those contemporaries who opposed Ehrlich's theory, and then by the new wave of immunochemists who would substitute for this selective theory one based on instruction by antigen (see later).

The answer that Ehrlich provides to this paradox is in fact not especially satisfying, but is perhaps the only possible statement that an implacably logical biologist could offer. "One may therefore rightly assume that these toxophile protoplasmic groups [receptors] in reality serve normal functions in the animal organism, and that they only incidentally and by pure chance possess the capacity to anchor themselves to this or that toxin." If antibodies are truly cell receptors (as Ehrlich firmly believes), and if they cannot have evolved to such foreign substances never normally encountered (as common sense dictates), then their apparent specificity for these substances *must by logic* arise from accidental crossreactions. Taken further, this leads inevitably to the conclusion that the atomic structure of the combining site (haptophore group) of every foreign toxins must be identical to that of some nutrient important to the normal physiology of the cell; this is what cross-reaction demands. This conclusion is logically forced, but is it reasonable? Ehrlich would surely not have questioned it, but it is curious that the implausibility of the argument was overlooked by those who opposed his side-chain theory.

There is another, even more subtle, problem with the Ehrlich formulation that seems to have been overlooked by its opponents. If the interaction of toxins with their receptors leads to the release of antitoxins into the blood, why does the interaction of essential nutrients with *their* receptors not lead to the similar release of antinutrient antibodies? Just as the one protects the cell from toxic action, so the other should "protect" it from its sustenance!

Ehrlich next provides an explanation for the inability of small molecules to induce an antibody response. He points out that not long after administration, toxins attach tightly to the tissues of the host and can neither be dissolved off nor readily neutralized *in situ*. This is because they have become tightly attached to their specific receptors (i.e., what would later be called "cell-bound" antibodies) But, by contrast, small molecules such as sugars, alkaloids, and aromatic amines can readily be removed from the tissues by appropriate solvents. This is because there is no receptor present to anchor them and thus no possibility to induce receptor proliferation (antibody formation).

Ehrlich then deals with the phenomenon of *natural immunity*. This, he claims, is due to the absence in certain species of the receptors required to anchor certain bacterial toxins, which would permit them to damage the cells to which they are attached. The dog, for example, presumably lacking receptors for ptomaines, is exempt from the disease that afflicts man, monkey, and rabbit, all of whom possess these ptomaine-receptors in abundance. Ehrlich also provides an explanation for what would later be called *natural antibodies*.[24] Noting that antitoxins have been observed in the blood of individuals not previously exposed to these agents, Ehrlich suggests that they are merely the receptors produced by the excessive action of those nutrients that cross react with the antitoxins in question.[25]

Ehrlich next presents the famous cartoons that take the reader pictorially step by step through his concept of the function of cell surface receptors, of immunological specificity, and of the process that leads to the production of circulating antibody (Fig. 6.1).[26] For the first time,[27] one was able literally to "see" the steps in the logical development of the side-chain theory. In cartoon 1 is represented a cell possessing receptors (side chains) for each of the external substances that the cell requires for its various functions. Note that Ehrlich represents each specificity with its own geometric design at the binding site, fitting together "as lock and key," designations that generations of immunologists would employ in their blackboard and lantern slide presentations of specific antigen-antibody interactions. In the second cartoon, a toxin is represented bound to its specific cell receptor, the only way that its (brush-border) toxophore group could exert its damaging effect. In cartoon 3, many toxin molecules are shown binding to their receptors, leading in 4 to an overcompensatory production of these.[28] The excess receptors are then shed from the cell, to appear as circulating antibody. It is these free antibodies in the blood that will thenceforth interact with and neutralize toxin before it can become anchored to the target cell, thus protecting the host from later exposure. But whereas many were convinced that they could "see" the materiality of the antibody in these pictures, Frederick Gay (Jules Bordet's student) would say of them, "They seem to have yielded an unfortunate sense of material stability to an incorrect explanation of the functions that they were meant to represent."[29]

By the time that he gave the Croonian Lecture, Ehrlich had responded to Jules Bordet's publication on immune hemolysis with some of his own experiments on the subject, performed with Julius Morgenroth. In concluding this lecture, he touched on some of these findings. When finally completed in 1901, these six

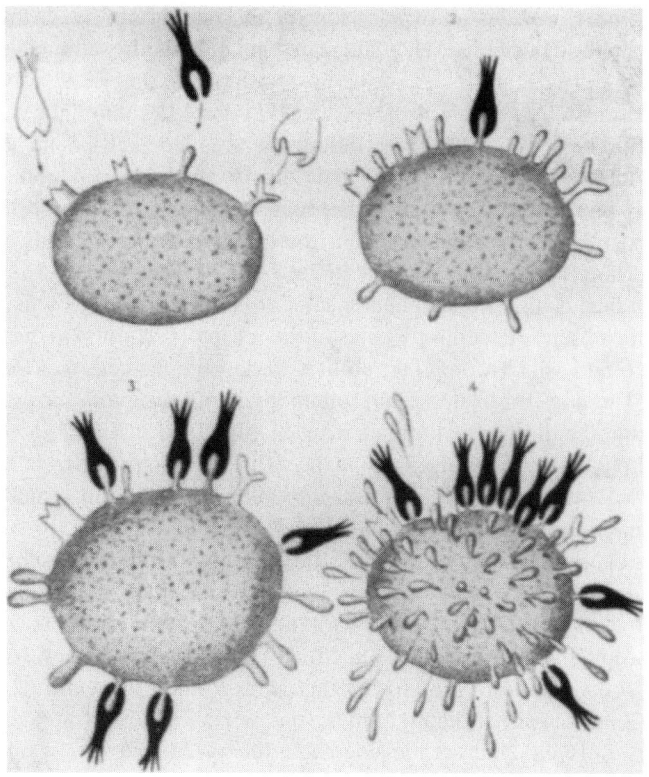

FIGURE 6.1   The diagrammatic representation of the side-chain theory. (1) The cell possesses
many receptors (antibodies) with different specificities; (2) The toxin molecule interacts with its specific receptor; (3) The neutralization of many identical receptors affects the cell; and (4) The cell over-
regenerates these receptors, casting the excess off into the blood. (After Ehrlich, note 22.)

reports would constitute some of his most important contributions to experimental immunology, and would incorporate important extensions of his side-chain
theory and his concept of the structure and function of antibodies. They, and additional publication that discuss the side-chain theory in the context of immune
hemolysis, will be discussed in detail in the next chapter.

THESIS, ANTITHESIS, AND SYNTHESIS

In the years that followed Ehrlich's publication of his theory, and especially after
its expansion and illustration in the Croonian Lecture, the implications of receptors
and specificity for biology and medicine were widely advertised. This was true
above all in Germany, where already Paul Ehrlich was regarded as one of its leading
scientists. Numerous books, pamphlets, and papers were written attesting to the

advantages gained from the application of the concepts to one or another field. Chapters could be found on "the side-chain theory in internal medicine," "the side-chain theory in obstetrics and gynecology," and so on and it was held that adherence to Ehrlich's tenets would solve most problems in preventive immunization.[30]

An interesting booklet appeared in 1908, authored by a Russian from Kharkov, Dr. P. Schatiloff, then working at the Institute for Research in Infectious Diseases in Bern, Switzerland. Schatiloff worried that Ehrlich's theory might not have been explained sufficiently and was unfairly deemed too difficult to grasp. He, Schatiloff, would present the theory in a more comprehensible form, emphsizing pedagogy rather than new research findings.[31] For this purpose, he employed cartoons that went even further than Ehrlich in picturing the numerous components and their interactions. As Cambrosio *et al.* point out,[32] Schatiloff's diagrams provide almost a Mendeleevian periodic table of immunological elements whose chemical combinations can almost be visualized. Perhaps the most impressive of Schatiloff's diagrams is his pictorial summary of all the active cells, the immunological reactants, and their possible combinations, as reproduced in Figure 6.2. Here is every type of receptor, every specificity, toxins, complements, and all of their combinations. It was assumed, apparently, that careful study of this schema and the accompanying tables would lead to a full understanding of all of contemporary immunology.

The Opponents

We noted in the last chapter that Ehrlich's ideas were opposed by both Jules Bordet and Svante Arrhenius. However, both these distinguished scientists payed little attention to Ehrlich's concept of how antibodies are formed, preferring to challenge him on his concept of the mechanism of their function. Bordet did object strenuously, however, to Ehrlich's cartoons, later referring to them as "puerile graphical representation"[33]—this despite Ehrlich's earlier caution that, "Needless to say, these diagrams must be regarded as quite apart from all morphologic considerations."[34]

In the forefront of opposition to Ehrlich's ideas was Max von Gruber, a Viennese hygienist working in Munich at the time of his polemical exchanges with Ehrlich. It was in Gruber's laboratory in 1896 that Herbert Durham had discovered the phenomenon of bacterial agglutination by antibody.[35] Although Gruber's attack on Ehrlich revolved primarily around the question of the nature of immunological specificity, his critical salvos were aimed at every aspect of Ehrlich's theories, not sparing his theory of antibody formation.

It will be recalled that in 1897, at the time that Ehrlich speculated on the receptor origins of circulating antibodies, only a few substances were known to stimulate the immune response. These were, almost without exception, toxins derived from bacterial or plant origin. But over the course of the next few years, many other substances of widely diverse origins were found to induce specific antibody formation. These included xenogeneic and isogeneic erythrocytes and other cell types, serum and egg proteins, and eventually even pollens and complex polysaccharides. Thus,

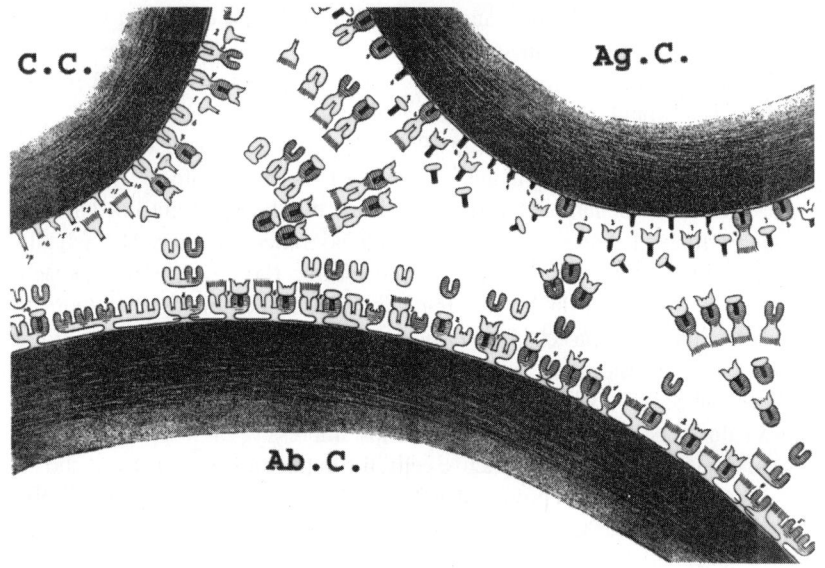

FIGURE 6.2   Schatiloff's attempt to summarize in a single cartoon the many cells, molecules, and processes involved in Ehrlich's side-chain interpretation of immunological functions. Ag.C. = antigenic cell; Ab.C. = antibody-forming cell; C.C. = complement-producing cell. (After Schatilloff, note 31.)

almost day by day, the growth of the immunological repertoire posed an increasingly strong challenge to Ehrlich's initial explanation of nutrient-receptor crossreactions with toxins.

Gruber recognized this paradox immediately, and did not hesitate to pose the questions that logically followed. How, he asked Ehrlich accusingly, is it possible to explain, even in chemical terms, the astonishingly large number of different specificities that the immune system was capable of producing?[36] How, from the point of view of Darwinian evolution, could all of these antibody specificities have arisen to antigens not in the normal environment? Obviously, Ehrlich's explanation of "accidental crossreactions" seemed to many no longer to be tenable.

There was another not quite so telling argument against Ehrlich's theory of antibody formation. Toxins were supposed to act only on those tissues that contained receptors permitting their attachment to the target cells—hence, only the tissues with these receptors should engage in antibody formation. Thus, neurotoxins such as tetanus toxin localize predominently in the brain, as might be expected from their physiological effects. However, most studies placed the site of formation of antibodies in the lymphatic tissues and bone marrow.[37] There were no reports of tetanus antitoxin formation in the central nervous system.

SELECTION GIVES WAY TO INSTRUCTION

The disclosure of the ever-increasing size of the immunological repertoire was the rock on which Ehrlich's theory of antibody formation[38] would founder. The full extent of the conceptual problem was pointed up by the report of Obermeyer and Pick that simple chemicals attached to a carrier protein would induce antibody formation specific for these simple structures.[39] If a specific antibody can be produced against any structure that can be synthesized in the organic chemistry laboratory, including those hitherto unknown in nature, Ehrlich's idea of cross-reaction with nutrients becomes highly implausible. While his receptor concept continued to influence the field of pharmacology,[40] it rapidly disappeared from view in considerations of the mechanism of antibody formation. Over the next several decades, it was mentioned in passing as of merely historical interest,[41] if it was mentioned at all.[42]

Following World War I, immunology, in its classical mode as a medical specialty concerned with infectious diseases, went into decline.[43] Serotherapy could not be generalized beyong diphtheria and tetanus, and new advances in preventive vaccines were few and far between. Interest shifted to more chemical pursuits, as exemplified by the work of Karl Landsteiner, John Marrack, and Michael Heidelberger. The emphasis in both investigation and in thought shifted from questions of biological mechanism to those of chemical structure and specificity. But the problem of an immense antibody repertoire persisted, and it should come as no surprise that if this conceptual vacuum were to be filled at all in the 1930s, it would take a chemical rather than a biological form.

Felix Haurowitz

It was understood by 1930 that proteins were composed of presumably random arrangements of the 20-odd amino acids, and that antibodies are globular proteins. If, as previously suggested, the information for antibody specificity could not possibly be inherent in the host, then it must perforce be carried in from outside, and only the antigen could play this instructive role. This idea was advanced independently and almost simultaneously by a number of different investigators,[44] but it assumed its most definitive form at the hands of Breinl and Haurowitz.[45] It is interesting that, like Ehrlich, Breinl and Haurowitz introduced their theory as an almost incidental addendum to a research report, in this case on the immunochemistry of hemoglobin. The theory was, for the period, elegantly simple. Antigen would be carried to the site of protein formation, where it would guide the synthesis of a unique sequence of amino acids, thus determining the specificity of the resulting antibody molecule. In fact, each antigen would act as a *template,* and in this manner provide the information necessary for the production of the unique specificity required to interact with that structural determinant.

Linus Pauling

The Breinl–Haurowitz instructive template theory was modified some years later by Linus Pauling,[46] when it became evident that the amino acid sequence of protein molecules might not be thoroughly random. Pauling suggested that the function of antigen was to order the unique folding of the amino acid chain on a *nascent* globulin molecule, thus forming for each antigen a complementary, three-dimensional combining site.

These instructionist theories, with their somewhat Lamarckian flavor, appealed to the immunochemists who dominated the field between the 1930s and 1950s. They appeared to solve the critical chemical problems posed by the data—the vastness of the repertoire and the fine specificity of the antigen–antibody interaction. Chemists, unlike biologists, are unconcerned with questions of Darwinian evolution; the molecules of the chemist, unlike those of the biologist, have no evolutionary history. In addition, the immunochemists chose to disregard the more biological aspects of the immune response, such as the anamnestic response and affinity maturation.

Macfarlane Burnet

So well entrenched was instruction during this period, and so well forgotten was Paul Ehrlich's theory, that even biologist Macfarlane Burnet could advance instructionist theories of antibody formation. Attempting to "biologize" the role of antigen, Burnet suggested in 1941 that antigen would induce specific *adaptive enzymes* that would then engage in the synthesis of antibody specific for the stimulating antigen.[47] Later, when the notion that enzymes might be adaptively modified fell out of favor, Burnet, ever in tune with the times, modified his theory to propose that antigen might impress the information for its specificity on the (?RNA) genome, on which *indirect template* antibody specifity could be molded during protein formation.[48] Perhaps the most significant contribution of Burnet's early theories was his suggestion that antibody formation is the product not only of the cells initially stimulated, *but of their descendents also.* We shall soon appreciate the importance of this concept of a role for cellular dynamics.

THE RETURN TO SELECTION

Two developments in the 1950s heralded the demise of instructionist theories of antibody formation. The first rested on new data on the mechanism of protein formation, especially on the finding that the information for all protein formation is encoded in a DNA genome. Francis Crick's "Central Dogma," that information can only move from DNA to RNA to protein and cannot originate in a protein, seemed to doom the concept of antigenic instruction. The second development lay in the underlying transition that was taking place from immunochemistry to immunobiology. A new generation of medically and biologically trained individuals became interested in such questions as the hightened booster antibody response, the origin of "natural" antibodies, transplantation immunology, immunodeficiency diseases, immunological tolerance, and autoimmunity. These were questions that challenged both the concepts and the practices of chemically oriented immunologists.

Niels Jerne

From this period of turbulent change came, in 1955, Niels Jerne's natural selection theory of antibody formation.[49] His concept was not far from that of Ehrlich, although the latter was not referenced in the paper. Jerne proposed that all possible specificities occur naturally in the host, and circulate as "natural antibodies." Antigen then *selects* from among that pool and is then transported by its specific antibody to the appropriate cell, in which black box and by mechanism unknown further production of the same specificity is stimulated. The theory proved valuable in three respects:

1. It explained the magnified booster response by suggesting an increase in production "efficiency"—Ehrlich had suggested this also.
2. It offered a solution to that purely biological paradox, the recently discovered phenomenon of immunological tolerance[50]—antibodies against self would by absorbed *in vivo* by their respective antigens, and thus would not be available to transport new antigen for further stimulation of anti-self response.
3. Curiously, Jerne's theory will probably be remembered, not so much for its intrinsic value, but rather for the fact that it stimulated Macfarlane Burnet to point his fertile imagination in a new direction.

Macfarlane Burnet's New Synthesis

In 1957, his reading of Jerne's provocative paper caused Burnet to put together the four critical elements that would determine his new theory of antibody formation:[51] (1) Jerne's (and Ehrlich's) idea of naturally occurring antibodies; (2) Ehrlich's idea of cell surface receptors; (3) Burnet's own recognition of the dynamics of cell proliferation; and (4) the concept of somatic mutation of DNA. This potent combination would help to explain, or at least begin to explain, most of the perplexing aspects of the immune response. As Burnet would later recall,

> It gradually dawned upon me that Jerne's selection theory would make real sense if cells produced a characteristic pattern of globulin for genetic reasons and were stimulated to proliferate by contact with the corresponding antigenic determinant. This would demand a receptor on the cell with the same pattern as the antibody and a signal resulting from contact of antigenic determinant and receptor that would initiate mitosis or other cellular reaction.[52]

Note the similarity of concept to Ehrlich's scheme: "characteristic pattern"; "receptor on the cell with the same pattern"; "initiate ... cellular reaction." Missing only were the more modern terms, "genetic," "signal," and "proliferation/mitosis." It is worth noting that the germ of the same idea was published independently that same year by David Talmage.[53]

Apparently Burnet was so unsure of his theory at the outset that he chose to publish it in a somewhat obscure Australian journal, rather than in one of his more customary prestigious outlets like *Nature*. However, the theory was so well received that Burnet felt free to expand on it and its consequences in a full book published in 1959.[54] Now, not only were all antibodies formed by the host under the direction of its own DNA, but they appear spontaneously as receptors on the surface membrane of lymphoid cells, one specificity per cell. The large repertoire is provided by the action of somatic mutational events on a more modest library of immunoglobulin genes. Finally, an antigen will *select* for activation only those cells that bear its corresponding receptors, resulting in their differentiation for active antibody formation and their clonal proliferation. Here was an explanation of most of the biological features of the immune response: the difference between primary and booster responses; the continued formation of antibody in the absence of antigen; and affinity maturation, due to minor somatic mutations during the course of repeated booster injections. Even the perplexing question of immunological tolerance was explained by the postulated elimination of anti-self clonal precursors during a critical period in fetal development.

Talmage and Lederberg

Burnet's clonal selection theory stimulated two papers that contributed important elaborations and theoretical support. In his contribution,[55] David Talmage not only expanded on the role of antigen selection and antigen-induced cell activation, but was the first of the selectionists to confront the problem of repertoire size. He emphasized that an immune serum may contain a very large number of cross-reacting antibodies (what we now call the *degeneracy* of the immune respoonse), and that its overall fine specificity might merely depend on the differing ratios of the several antibodies present. Thus, the basic repertoire might not number in the millions, but rather only in the thousands, a not unreasonable number to have stored in the vertebrate genome. Joshua Lederberg, for his part, brought the prestige of a Nobel Prize-winning geneticist to a discussion of some of the fine points of the theory.[56] Immunological specificity is determined by a unique primary sequence of amino acids, determined by a unique sequence of nucleotides in a "gene for globulin synthesis." Lederberg went on to suggest that a high rate of spontaneous *and random* somatic mutation of DNA in this immunoglobulin gene, not only during the fetal period as Burnet had suggested, but throughout life, would readily account for the diversity of the antibody repertoire. This emphasis on the overriding importance of somatic mutation in the generation of immunological diversity would result in a decades-long debate between those who believed that most of the information is stored in the germline (the multigene protagonists) and those who believed that only a very limited number of germline genes acted on by mutations explains the repertoire (the pauci-gene advocates).[57]

EHRLICH REVISITED

Every theory from the past must be measured, not in terms of what is known today, but in the context of the state of contemporary knowledge. Even ideas that today seem naive or even groundless may, at the time, not only have appeared to be correct, but may even have served broader heuristic functions. In the case of Paul Ehrlich's side-chain theory of antibody formation, we view 100 years later a theory that was essentially correct in its most important elements. These include the notion that antibodies are naturally occurring substances, that they serve as *receptors* on the surface of the cells that form them, and that they constitute the targets of antigenic *selection* for expanded antibody formation. Of course, Ehrlich was wrong in attributing this capacity to all cells; he could not have known at the time that it is restricted to lymphocyte lineages, or that the mechanism depends on a complicated signal transduction that would act on an even more complicated genetic mechanism involving the variable assembly of minigene segments. Finally, Ehrlich's suggestion that the original function of these receptors had to do with cell nutrition was imaginative, but ultimately erroneous. Only with the ability to sequence the amino acids of proteins in the search for homologies has it been shown that antibody receptors probably have evolved from more primitive cell membrane adhesion or recognition molecules important for the differentiation and maintenance of the integrity of all multicellular organisms.[58]

What is interesting about Ehrlich's receptor theory is how productive it was at the time in explaining the specificity of immunological interactions, and of drug and enzyme reactions as well. But the general concept appears to have disappeared from view for over half a century. One searches in vain for signs that it directly influenced Jerne or Burnet in their formulation of theories so akin to that of Ehrlich's original one. Moreover, in these times when almost every physiological process from taste buds and olfaction to the workings of hormones and endorphins is viewed as depending on receptors, it is difficult to find any thread that links these present concepts back to Ehrlich. Apparently some ideas must be discovered and then rediscovered, each in its own time and context.

NOTES AND REFERENCES

1. Thucidides, *The Peloponnesian War* (Crawley Transl.), New York, Modern Library, 1934, p. 112.
2. Rhazes, *A Treatise on the Smallpox and Measles* (W.A. Greenhill transl.), London, Sydenham Society, 1848.
3. Girolamo Fracastoro, *De Contagione et Contagionis Morbis et Eorum Curatione* (W.C. Wright transl.), New York, Putnam, 1930, pp. 60–63.
4. Carmichael, A.E. and Silverstein, A.M., *J. Hist. Med. Allied Sci.* 42:147, 1987, have speculated that perhaps only a mild form of smallpox, akin to *Variola minor,* existed in Europe prior to the seventeenth century.
5. Drake, J., *Anthropologia Nova, or, a New System of Anatomy,* London, 1717, vol. I, p. 25.
6. Fuller, T., *Exanthematologia: or an Attempt to give a rational account of Eruptive Fevers,* London, 1730, p. 175 ff.

7. Pasteur, L., Chamberland, C., and Roux, E., *C.R. Acad. Sci.* 90:239, 1880.
8. Metchnikoff, I., *Virchows Archiv.* 96:177, 1884. The theory is broadly fleshed out in Metchnikoff's *Immunity in the Infectious Diseases,* New York, Macmillan, 1905.
9. The violent debate between predominently French "cellularists" and predominently German "humoralists" is discussed in detail by Silverstein, A.M., *A History of Immunology,* New York, Academic Press, 1989, pp. 38–58.
10. Nuttall, G., *Z. Hygiene* 4:353, 1888; Buchner, H., *Zentralbl. Bakteriol.* 6:561, 1889.
11. Behring E. and Kitasato, S., *Deutsch. med. Wochenschr.* 16:1113, 1890; see also Behring, E. and Wernicke, E., *Z. Hygiene* 12:10, 45, 1892.
12. Buchner, H., *Münch. med. Wochenschr.* 40:449, 480, 482, 1893.
13. Later template theories of antibody formation (see later) would demand the persistence of antigen for continued antibody formation. Even as late as the 1960s, Dan Campbell, student of Linus Pauling and still a firm believer in Pauling's template theory, would continue the search for persisting antigen; see Campbell, D.H. and Garvey, J.S., "Retained antigen and immune mechanisms," *Adv. Immunol.* 3:261, 1963.
14. Roux E. and Vaillard, L., *Ann. Inst. Pasteur* 7:65, 1893; Knorr, A., *Münch. med. Wochenschr.* 45:321, 362, 1898.
15. See also the history of receptor theory in pharmacology by Parascandola, J. and Jasensky, R., *Bull. Hist. Med.* 48:199, 1974, and Silverstein, A.M., "Paul Ehrlich's passion: The origins of his receptor immunology," *Cell. Immunol.* 194:213, 1999.
16. Ehrlich, P., *Klin. Jahrbuch* 6:299, 1897; English translation in *The Collected Papers of Paul Ehrlich,* London, Pergamon, 1956–1960, vol. II, p. 114 (henceforth *Collected papers*). These effects are the hallmarks of the kinetics of chemical reactions.
17. Ehrlich, *Collected Papers,* note 16, vol. II, p. 114.
18. Weigert, C., *Verh. Ges. Deutsch. Naturforsch. Aerzte.* 68:121, 1896.
19. Ehrlich, P., *Deutsch. med. Wochenschr.* 24:597, 1898; English version in *Trans. Jenner Inst, Prevent. Med.* 1899; *Collected Papers* vol. II, pp. 126–133 and 134–142.
20. Ehrlich's speech has never been published in its original form, but a translation into French was made from the manuscript by a Dr. Villaret, and published in *Semaine Méd. Paris* 19:411, 1899.
21. Belfanti, S. and Carbone, T., *G.R. Acad. Torino* 46:321, 1898; Bordet, J., *Ann. Inst. Pasteur* 12:688, 1899.
22. Ehrlich, P., *Proc. Roy. Soc. London,* 66:424, 1900; *Collected Papers* vol. II, pp. 178–195.
23. Ehrlich, note 22, *Collected Papers,* vol. II, pp. 183–184.
24. Ehrlich, note 22, *Collected Papers,* vol. II, pp. 188–189.
25. This suggestion would foreshadow the conclusion that many "natural antibodies" (e.g., blood group isoagglutinins, etc.) are formed against exogenous cross-reacting determinants primarily from the gastrointestinal tract. See, e.g., S. Boyden, *Advances Immunol.* 5:1, 1966.
26. The significance, both discursive and epistemological, of Ehrlich's pictorializations is provided by Cambrosio, A., Jacobi, D. and Keating, P., "Ehrlich's 'beautiful pictures' and the controversial beginnings of immunological imagery," in *Usages de l'Image au XIXe Siècle,* S. Michaud *et al.,* eds., Paris, Créaphis, 1992.
27. Ehrlich had earlier anticipated these cartoons in a letter to his cousin Carl Weigert, described in B. Heyman's history of the side-chain theory, *Klin. Wochenschr.* 7:1257, 1305, 1938.
28. There is a certain illogic in this presentation, not addressed either by Ehrlich or by his detractors. With so many toxin molecules on the cell presumably able to exert their damaging effect, how then has the cell time to produce so much antibody over time?
29. Gay, F., *Agents of disease and host resistance,* Springfield, Charles Thomas, 1935, p. 379. Gay, of course, followed his mentor Bordet in believing in an *unstable* physical interaction of antigen with antibody—see Chapter 7.
30. See, e.g., Aschoff, L., *Ehrlichs Seitenkettentheorie und ihre Anwendung auf die kunstlichen Immunisierungsprozesse,* Jena, Gustav Fischer, 1902; Römer, P., *Die Ehrlichsche Seitenkettentheorie und ihre Bedeutung für die medizinischen Wissenschaften,* Vienna, Hölder, 1904.

31. Schatiloff, P., *Die Ehrlichsche Seitenkettentheorie: Erläutert und Bildlich Dargestellt,* Jena, Gustav Fischer, 1908.
32. Cambrosio *et al.,* note 26.
33. Bordet, J., *Traité de l'Immunité dans les Maladies Infectieuses,* Paris, Masson, 1920 p. 504.
34. Ehrlich, note 22, *Collected Papers,* vol. II, p. 187.
35. von Gruber, M. and Durham, H.E., *Münch. med. Wochenschr.* 43:285, 1896.
36. von Gruber, M., *Münch. med. Wochenschr.* 48:1214, 1901. Others asked the same question; see Buchner, H., *Münch. med. Wochenschr.* 47:277, 1900; Hopf, L., *Immunität und Immunisierung,* Tübingen, Pietzker, 1902, p. 89.
37. See, e.g., Pfeiffer R. and Marx, E., *Z. Hygiene* 27:272, 1898; Wassermann, A., *Berlin klin. Wochenschr.* 35:209, 1898; Castellani, A., *Z. Hygiene* 37:381, 1901.
38. A detailed history of theories of antibody formation will be found in Silverstein, *A History of Immunology,* note 9, pp. 59–86.
39. Obermeyer, F. and Pick, E.P., *Wien. klin. Wochenschr.* 19:327, 1906. Later, Pick would publish an encyclopedic summary (in Kolle and Wassermann's *Handbuch der pathogenen Mikroorganismen,* 2nd ed., vol. I, Jena, Gustav Fischer, 1912, pp. 685–868) of the many synthetic chemicals (called *haptens*) against which specific antibodies could be formed. Karl Landsteiner would later put this approach to such good use in his *Specificity of Serological Reactions,* New York, Dover Reprint, 1962.
40. Parascandola and Jasensky, note 15.
41. Zinsser, H., *Infection and Resistance,* New York, Macmillan, 1914; Karsner, H.T. and Ecker, E.E., *The Principles of Immunology,* Philadelphia, Lippincott, 1921; Topley, W.W.C. and Wilson, G.S., *The Principles of Bacteriology and Immunity,* Baltimore, William Wood, 1929. Topley, in his *An Outline of Immunity* (Baltimore, William Wood, 1935, p. 82) indicates that while the side-chain theory "forms a good working model of our current views [of the antigen-antibody interaction] … it suggests a theory of the formation of antibodies which must be rejected."
42. Muir, R., *Studies on Immunity,* London, Oxford University Press, 1909; Gideon Wells, H., *The Chemical Aspects of Immunity,* New York, Chemical Catalog, 1929; Marrack, J.R., *The Chemistry of Antigens and Antibodies,* London, H.M. Printing Office, 1934.
43. For a general discussion of the disciplinary phases through which immunology passed, see Silverstein, A.M., *Cell. Immunol.* 132:515, 1991. In 1935, Topley (*An Outline,* note 41, p. v) could say, "It is probable that no subject in the medical curriculum is, at the moment, in a less satisfactory position than that to which we attach the label *Immunity.* It is a hybrid creature, not quite sure of its true affiliations."
44. Topley, W.W.C., *J. Path. Bact.* 33:341, 1930; Alexander, J., *Protoplasma* 14:296, 1931; and Mudd, S., *J. Immunol.* 23:423, 1932.
45. Breinl F. and Haurowitz, F., *Z. Physiol. Chem.* 192:45, 1930. See also Haurowitz, F., *Nature (London)* 205:847, 1965. Felix Haurowitz was one of the very few who clung tenaciously to an instructive theory of antibody formation even after the apparent success of Burnet's clonal selection theory.
46. Pauling, L., *J. Am. Chem. Soc.* 62:2643, 1940; *Science* 92:77, 1940.
47. Burnet, F.M., *The Production of Antibodies,* New York, Macmillan, 1941.
48. Burnet, F.M. and Fenner, F., *The Production of Antibodies* 2nd ed., New York, Macmillan, 1949.
49. Jerne, N.K., *Proc. Nat. Acad. Sci. US,* 41:849, 1955.
50. Burnet and Fenner in 1949 (note 48) had suggested the existence of the phenomenon of immunological tolerance, and Billingham, R.E., Brent, L., and Medawar, P.B., proved the reality of tolerance experimentally (*Nature (London)* 172:603, 1953), for which Burnet and Medawar shared the Nobel Prize in 1960.
51. Burnet, F.M., *Austral. J. Sci.* 20:67, 1957.
52. Burnet, F.M., "The impact of ideas on immunology," *Cold Spring Harbor Symp. Quant. Biol.* 32:1–8, 1967, p. 2.
53. D. Talmage, *Ann. Rev. Med.* 8:239, 1957.
54. Burnet, F.M., *The Clonal Selection Theory of Antibody Formation.* London, Cambridge University Press, 1959.

55. Talmage, D., *Science* 129:1643, 1959.
56. Lederberg, J., *Science* 129:1649, 1959.
57. The history of this debate, and the final compromise solution, is well delineated in Kindt, T.J. and Capra, J.D., *The Antibody Enigma,* New York, Plenum Press, 1984. See also Podolsky, S.H. and Tauber, A.I., *The Generation of Diversity: Clonal Selection Theory and the Rise of Molecular Immunology,* Cambridge MA, Harvard University Press, 1997.
58. Edelman, G.M., *Immunol. Rev.* 100:11, 1987.

7

IMMUNE HEMOLYSIS: BORDET CHALLENGES EHRLICH

Against that positivism which stops before phenomena, say-
ing 'there are only facts,' I should say: 'No, it is precisely facts
that do not exist, only interpretations.'

Nietzsche

In 1898 came the report from Paris of a new discovery in immunity research that would become one of the most useful technologies in the armamentarium of the immunologist. Jules Bordet, a young assistant to Elie Metchnikoff at the Pasteur Institute, reported that red cells could be hemolyzed by the combined action of two substances, one heat-stable and the other heat-labile.[1] The phenomenon had earlier been reported by Belfanti and Carbone,[2] but it would be Bordet who would fully realize the important implications and powerful applications of this approach. He would not only use the system as a vehicle to challenge Ehrlich's concepts of how antigens and antibodies interact, but would later demonstrate how complement fixation may be utilized to test for antigens or antibodies.[3] This approach would soon be adapted by August Wassermann for the diagnosis of syphilis,[4] the founding methodology of the new field of serology.

The heuristic value of the phenomenon of immune hemolysis (and of the related hemagglutination) would soon extend far beyond the diagnostic complement fixation test.[5] It would assume great importance in blood typing[6] and thence in blood transfusion and in anthropological studies;[7] in defining the first of many autoimmune hemolytic diseases, paroxysmal cold hemoglobinuria;[8] and it would eventually provide the basis for the hemolytic plaque assay technic of Jerne and Nordin,[9] which played so important a role in defining the cell dynamics of the immune response.

The discovery of immune hemolysis was immediately recognized not to be a unique phenomenon, but merely another manifestation of a more general type of reaction—the destruction of a cell through the mediation of specific antibody and complement. It will be recalled that, in 1895, Richard Pfeiffer had reported that cholera vibrios injected into the peritoneal cavity of immune guinea pigs are rapidly destroyed,[10] a reaction that Elie Metchnikoff demonstrated could also be observed *in vitro*.[11] Bordet was soon able to show[12] that bacteriolysis depends on the action of two substances, a thermostable factor in the serum of immunized animals (antibody) and the thermolabile factor that had earlier been discovered and named *Alexin* by Hans Buchner.[13] Bordet would always prefer the term alexine to Ehrlich's *Komplement;* since the latter term has survived to this day, we will use it (or rather its anglicized version *complement*) henceforth unless "alexine" is required for the argument. Thus, immune hemolysis and immune bacteriolysis were similar phenomena, dependent on the workings of the same two substances.

THE FIRST ROUND

Bordet Describes Immune Hemolysis

Bordet published his first paper on immune hemolysis in October 1898. He recalled to the reader Pfeiffer's observation on the killing of cholera vibrios, and his own demonstration of the requirement for two substances, one specific and thermostable and the other nonspecific and thermolabile. Now he refers to observations that the serum of certain animals possesses the ability to agglutinate the erythrocytes of other species and wonders about the possible analogy with the cholera vibrio phenomenon. He immunizes guinea pigs intraperitoneally with defibrinated rabbit blood, and can show that the fresh antiserum causes the agglutination and then the hemolysis of rabbit red cells, but only agglutination is seen if the serum is preheated to 55° C. However, fresh serum (either rabbit or guinea pig) will restore the power to hemolyze. Whereas the specificity of the antiserum for the species of red cells used for immunization may be demonstrated, Bordet shows that the action of the complement is not only nonspecific, but that a given complement can function in *any* antibody-erythrocyte system.

At this point, just a year after the publication of Ehrlich's side-chain theory, Bordet makes no mention of it. He does not discuss mechanism explicitly, restricting the report to phenomenological observations, with one interesting exception. Since the response to erythrocytes (which pose no threat) is identical to that against cholera vibrios (which pose a grand threat), Bordet concludes that the immune response cannot have arisen solely "to serve for defense against the microbe, any more than phagocytosis, the pivot of immunity, owes its existence and its *raison d'être* to a fight against microbes."[14] In paying his obligatory respects to the phagocytic theory of his chief Metchnikoff, Bordet concludes that immunity is nothing other than a particular case of intracellular digestion, a primordial function that would have existed even had there been no pathogenic organisms in the world.

Ehrlich Takes Up the Challenge

It is well known that Paul Ehrlich was an avid reader of the medical literature from all over the world, especially in the area of his current interests. He would have put high on his reading list the immunologically oriented *Annales de l'Institut Pasteur,* in which Bordet published his studies. The challenge to his side-chain theory implicit in Bordet's report could not go unanswered; it stimulated an immediate reaction from Ehrlich. Without delay, he assigned to his assistant Julius Morgenroth the task of repeating and extending Bordet's observations. Having at hand a quantity of goat anti-sheep blood, they were able within only 3 months to publish their initial results.[15] This report was intended to neutralize any challenge implicit in Bordet's report and to lend further confirmation to the validity of the side-chain theory.

In typical Ehrlich fashion, the first experiments sought to define the quantitative aspects of the phenomenon of immune hemolysis, by titrating the antiserum against a *dilute* suspension of defibrinated blood. In the process they found that, contrary to Bordet's report that hemolysis (of concentrated suspensions) is preceded by hemagglutination, in their hands (using more dilute reagents) agglutination and hemolysis were seemingly unrelated. From this they suggested that the agglutinating antibody and the hemolysing antibody are separate substances, a view that would later encompass all the secondary manifestations of antigen–antibody interactions. This view held sway until Hans Zinsser's *unitarian theory* of antibody action[16] becamed generally accepted some two to three decades later. They did confirm, however, Bordet's finding that two substances are required for hemolysis to proceed—one thermostable and the other thermolabile. Significantly, however, they chose not to employ Bordet's terminology of a "specific material in serum that renders [the cells] sensitive to the influence of the bactericidal substance" (later his *substance sensibilisatrice*) and *alexine;* they would employ the terms *immune-body* and *addiment.*

Ehrlich and Morgenroth now propose that application of the principles of the side-chain theory should shed light on the mechanism of hemolysis. Since the formation of any antibody must follow the attachment to cells of its stimulating antigen, they predict that the immune-body responsible for hemolysis should bind to the target erythrocytes. This they are able to demonstrate by absorbing the heated immune serum (heated to destroy its lytic ability) with sheep blood, and showed that after centrifugation of the mixture, all hemolytic antibody has been removed. Moreover, the sedimented red cells may be completely hemolyzed by the further addition of fresh serum. *"As a result of these experiments, therefore, and in conformity with the side-chain theory, we must assume that the immune-body possesses a specific haptophore group which anchors it to the blood-cells of the sheep* [their italics]."[17]

They then demonstrate that sheep red cells alone do not fix addiment, but that fixation of the antibody to the sheep cells in the cold carries along small amounts of fixed addiment, leaving the majority of it in the supernatant fluid. Interpreting these data in the context of the side-chain theory, they conclude that,

> The explanation of these phenomena presents no difficulties. It must be assumed that under certain circumstances the immune-body and the addiment enter into loose, readily dissociated chemical combination. ... On the other hand, the affinity existing between blood-cells and immune-body must be very strong, for these combine completely even in the cold ... the immune-body represents a link which ties addiment to the red blood-cells and subjects these to the action of the addiment.[18]

This is typical Ehrlich; all interactions, whether of weak or strong affinity, are chemical and involve specific atomic groupings. Thus, it is logical to assign to the hemolytic antibody two combining (haptophore) groups, one for the red cell (or bacterium) and the other for the addiment. In the same fashion, logic requires that the addiment possess two groupings also, a haptophore group for binding to antibody and another that carries the postulated enzyme (ferment) function responsible for destroying the red cell.

Here is the first structural modification of the side-chain theory to fit new facts; previous modifications had only required components of different binding affinities. The "simple" antitoxins described initially had but a single combining site for toxin. But the cell, being so much larger, requires a more complicated antibody molecule not only to fix to it, but also to mediate its destruction—thus the more complex hemolytic and bacteriolytic antibodies.

Bordet on Agglutination

In March 1899, Bordet published a lengthy review of theories of agglutination.[19] Although it does not bear directly on the dispute over immune hemolysis, we include it here in part for completeness and in part because in this paper Bordet draws two conclusions of far-reaching importance to the young field of immunology.

The main purpose of this review is to consider (and reject) a number of theories advanced to explain why microorganisms agglutinate when treated with specific antisera. In marshaling his arguments, Bordet shows that the phenomenon is a general one, since it also encompasses the agglutination of erythrocytes. He goes further and suggests that the precipitin reaction reported by Kraus[20] (involving such antigens as bacterial culture supernatants and even milk) is identical in mechanism to agglutination. He then repeats forcefully an earlier conclusion—the immune response must not be interpreted teleologically. It is a general physiological mechanism. "It is not with the aim of defending itself that the organism elaborates these injurious substances [antibacterial antibodies]. It simply brings into play against the microbes preexisting functional capabilities."

The second important point made by Bordet emerges from his demonstration that fixation of antibody to the cell and its agglutination are separate events. Taken together with the observation that fixation of hemolytic antibody to the red cell is independent of the subsequent hemolysis mediated by complement, and the apparent similarity of agglutination and precipitation, Bordet advances here a unitarian concept of antibody function some quarter-century before Zinsser.

THE SECOND ROUND

Bordet's Second Report on Hemolysis

In April 1899, Bordet expanded on his earlier study of hemagglutination and hemolysis in a second report.[21] We will explore this contribution in some detail, since it provided more detailed and specific targets for Ehrlich to contest. In this report, Bordet asks two questions: (1) Is there a basic difference between anti-erythrocyte and anti-bacterial sera? and (2) What is the relationship between the serum of a normal animal and that of an immunized animal? In his initial experiments, Bordet observes for the first time in the literature that only the blood of different species can stimulate an immune response; rabbit erythrocytes injected into the rabbit produce no agglutinating or hemolytic activity against rabbit cells.

Bordet repeats his earlier demonstration of the production of agglutinating and hemolyzing anti-erythrocyte antibodies, and shows that they may be passively administered to normal controls, conferring on the recipients the same qualities (albeit somewhat diluted) that were possessed by the immunized donor. He shows again the role played by complement in the hemolytic process, and that *any* complement, either from normal or immunized animals, will suffice. Thus, "One has no reason to suppose ... that the injection of active [immune] serum into a control animal will result in the secretion of a special dissolving alexine different from that found in control serum."[22] This observation will become the basis of a controversy between Ehrlich and Bordet on whether there is only a single nonspecific complement or a multiplicity of specific complements. We shall return to this question.

Bordet then proceeds to demonstrate once again the specificity of these antisera, showing, for example, that rabbit anti-chicken red cells do not affect guinea pig red cells. More convincing, and making yet another important immunological point, is Bordet's demonstration that absorption of a heated antiserum with the erythrocytes against which it has been formed will deplete the serum of all agglutinating and hemolytic capability. The red cells fix the the antibody (Bordet does not use this term; he prefers "the active substances") *avidly,* and they cannot be washed off. Bordet concludes with the statement that will characterize thenceforth his position and will excite the strong opposition of Paul Ehrlich,

> Such facts seem to prove clearly that this special substance, heat resistant, found in the serum of vaccinated [animals], and which permits the energetic dissolving action of alexine, *acts on the cells themselves,* to affect them directly and *to sensitize them* to the action of alexine [his italics].[23]

He also points out that there is no interaction between the alexine and the antibody, and that these coexist in an immune serum with no effect on one another. Further on, Bordet would express his thought more precisely: *"the specific sera contain a sensitizing substance* ['substance sensibilisatrice'] *which renders the cell or the microbe susceptible to be attacked by the alexine"* [his italics].[24] Note that Bordet refuses thus far to employ the Ehrlich term antibody (*Antikörper* = *anticorps*), and that while recognizing the tight binding of antibody to antigen, assigns it the function of merely preparing the cell for the destructive action of the complement.

Bordet then reports that the normal sera of most species possess agglutinins and hemolysins for the red cells of other species, in greater or lesser amounts; following immunization, these appear to be increased in amount and apparently also in their intrinsic activity. This leads Bordet to the "quite natural idea" that the properties acquired by the organism following immunization represent merely "the perfection, the *exaltation* of preexisting abilities."[25] Here is the prelude to an idea that both he and Karl Landsteiner[26] would later champion— that Ehrlich was wrong in suggesting that antibody of a single affinity was produced throughout. They would maintain that the effect of antigen is to further sharpen the specificity of the antibodies produced, an idea that sounds surprisingly like the modern concept of *affinity maturation.*

Ehrlich's Second Hemolysin Paper

In May 1899, Ehrlich and Morgenroth publish their second communication on hemolysins.[27] This is devoted, in the main, to confirming with better goat anti-sheep red cell sera the results obtained in the previous publication. In addition, they wish to argue the validity of their interpretation of the phenomenon and, for the first time, challenge Bordet's implicit interpretation. They repeat their earlier experiments that purport to show that hemolytic antibody has two combining sites, one for the red cell and another for their "addiment," and that the function of antibody is to *transport* the addiment to the cell surface, where it can act to destroy the cell. To point up their conceptual differences with Bordet, they now introduce a new nomenclature whose terms are semantically laden with implications about mechanism.[28] To counter Bordet's suggestion that hemolytic antibody functions as a "sensitizer," they introduce the name *Zwischenkörper* (the "body between," that connects the complement and the cell; they would later use the term *Ambozeptor* to imply the same process). Where Bordet employed the neutral term *alexine,* Ehrlich and Morgenroth introduce the new word *Komplement,* implying again that the substance acts with, or complements, the action of antibody.

To further highlight their differences with Bordet's interpretation that antibody "sensitizes" the red cell for the action of complement, they deride Bordet's metaphor, which suggests that the antibody acts "to change the structure of a lock, so as to permit the ready introduction of one or several keys which earlier could not enter, or did so only with difficulty."[29] But, they say, in this "mechanical conception," keys do not jump into a lock of their own accord, they require a driving force, which is "the chemical affinity between the fitting groups." Here are the contrasting views that will define the Bordet–Ehrlich dispute henceforth—the one involving physical forces and structural modifications, and the other defined by the affinity of chemical binding of complementary stereochemical structures.

Among the experiments reported in this paper are several whose interpretation would cause appreciable confusion in the years to come. First, there was the observation of a "heat-stable" complement. It will be recalled that heating normal serum at 56°C for 30 minutes will destroy its ability to mediate immune hemolysis when added with antiserum to a red cell suspension. But when Ehrlich and Morgenroth demonstrated that red cells could absorb antibody from heated serum in the cold without suffering damage, they measured this absorption by showing that the sensitized cells could then be hemolyzed by the addition of fresh (complement-rich) serum. But the same cells could apparently be lysed also by certain heated sera whose complement should have been inactivated. Under the impression that complement is a single entity, one had to conclude that some complements are heat-labile while others are heat-stable; it would be several decades before it was realized that complement is a complex mixture of labile and stable constituents that act in succession to cause hemolysis.[30]

The next complication arose from the view that hemolytic antibody is a "toxin" for the red cells, analogous to diphtheria or tetanus toxins. Thus, it should be possible to produce a specific anti-hemolysin, analogous to specific diphtheria or tetanus antitoxins. Therefore, goat anti-rabbit erythrocyte serum was injected into rabbits in an attempt to form this antibody. The results seemed convincing. Mixing the immune rabbit serum with the goat hemolytic serum not only prevented its hemolytic action against rabbit cells, it protected the cells of other species as well. It appeared logical to conclude that every serum contains a multiplicity of hemolytic antibodies, each able to excite the production of its corresponding antibodies.

Looking back, it strikes us as curious that researchers of that time could use blood or serum and disregard the presence of all constituents but the one in which they were interested. If red cells were required, then whole defibrinated blood was used; if sera were employed for their antibody or complement activity, then the presence of a multiplicity of other antigenic substances was ignored. It could not be imagined at the time that immunization with a serum (or whole blood) would induce the formation of antibodies against a variety of serum proteins, the interaction of each of these able to fix complement and interfere with the hemolytic test under consideration. We shall see further on how this misunderstanding would result in attempts to produce not only "anti-hemolysins," but also "anti-complements," leading to some extremely complex theoretical constructs.

The final complication arose from the demands of the side-chain theory for specificity when the binding groups of two substances interact. Thus, if the binding of antibody to antigen is specific, so ought the (looser) binding of complement to antibody, since haptophore binding groups were supposed to function here also. But this implies that each different hemolytic antibody should have its own specific complement; this factor is only hinted at in this communication, but it will play a larger role in further experiments and debates. It also provided the basis on which Ehrlich and Morgenroth expressed wonder that complement from a guinea pig can assist the function of a dog hemolytic antibody!

Ehrlich's Croonian Lecture

On March 22, 1900, Ehrlich presented the prestigious Croonian Lecture before the Royal Society of London.[31] He devotes the greater part of the lecture to his work with diphtheria toxin and to the side-chain theory (see Chapters 5 and 6), but refers at the end to immune hemolysis and to Bordet's and his own studies with Morgenroth. Once again, he emphasizes the chemical nature of the haptophore groups and that hemolytic antibody has two binding sites—one for the erythrocyte antigen and the other for complement. For its part, the complement molecule is also assigned two groupings, one to bind to antibody and the second to exercise its enzymatic/lytic activity. For the first time, Ehrlich illustrates his concepts with a set of cartoons (Fig. 7.1) that include his ideas about hemolytic antibody and complement, and that will influence the thinking of a generation of immunologists.

THE THIRD ROUND

Bordet Summarizes His Position

In May 1900, Jules Bordet published an extensive summary of the current knowledge of hemolytic antibodies, their anti-antibodies, and of the theories of their action.[32] By this time he would undoubtedly have seen Ehrlich's Croonian Lecture and have had full opportunity to consider all aspects of the first two communications on the subject by Ehrlich and Morgenroth. Bordet must at this point have been offended by his treatment at their hands: they had questioned his priority in the discovery of immune hemolysis by crediting Belfanti and Carbone with the discovery (see note 2); they seemed to take credit for the demonstration of the specificity of lytic antibodies; they insisted on the multiplicity of complements; and they appeared to trivialize Bordet's pioneering work on immune hemolysis by introducing a new terminology and asserting that everything could be explained in terms of Ehrlich's side-chain theory.

Thus, it is highly significant that the usually calm and generous Bordet reviews the entire field of immune hemolysis and mentions Ehrlich and Morgenroth only once! This reference occurs in a relatively minor context, and is presented as an experimental finding that "appears as a remarkable confirmation of this notion established by us several years earlier." Otherwise Bordet will, in effect, ostracize Ehrlich. He will not even mention Ehrlich's claims to priority or his theories in order to contest them—he will merely show that "someone else" should be credited with this-or-that finding or that a certain result could only be explained by an interpretation clearly opposed to the Ehrlich view. No one in the field reading this contribution could fail to appreciate that it was really an attack on Ehrlich by someone who felt ill used and unappreciated, but who was perhaps too polite to make explicit accusations.[33]

In this contribution, Bordet establishes at the very outset his priority in the discovery of the phenomenon of immune hemolysis. He reviews his earlier work

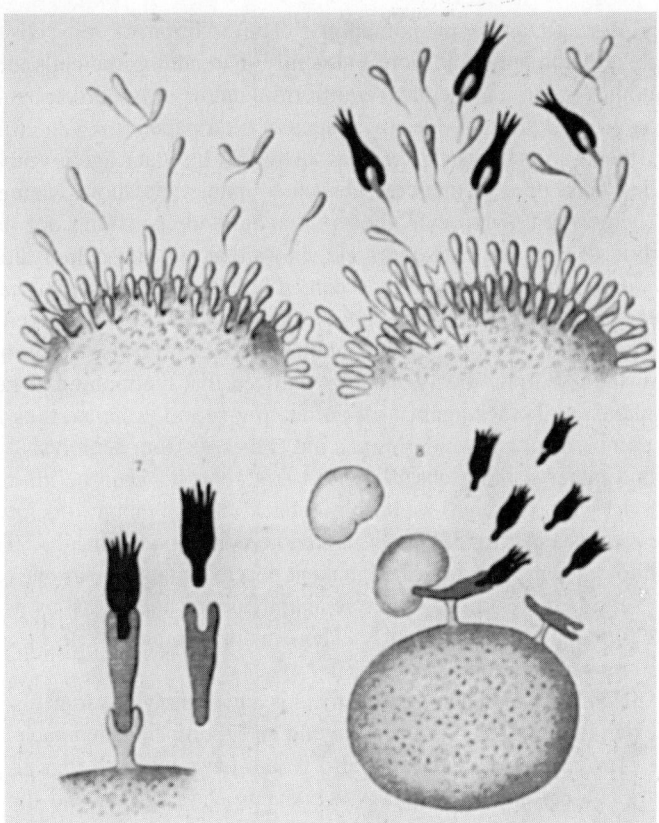

FIGURE 7.1   The side-chain theory and the structure of the components. (5) Receptors (anti-toxic antibodies) are cast off by the cell; (6) In the blood, they act to neutralize further exposure to toxins; (7) Hemolytic antibody, however, must have two combining sites, one for the cell antigen and one for complement; (8) To serve the more general function of nutrition, some receptors must carry combining sites for the enzymes which predigest the large molecule nutrient, permitting its entry into the cell. (After Ehrlich, note 31.)

showing the requirement for two components: a heat stable *substance sensibil-isatrice* and a thermolabile *alexine*. He even insists that his original system, involving guinea pig anti-rabbit erythrocytes and guinea pig complement, provides the best vehicle for these studies (Ehrlich and Morgenroth had used a goat anti-sheep system). He then reviews the principal phenomenology of immune hemolysis, most of whose points prove to be contradictions of Ehrlich's claims (although as indicated, the latter are never cited). Thus, Bordet shows that there is but a single nonspecific complement, active in both bacteriolysis and hemolysis. He shows that complement is not fixed until the red cell is "sensitized" by the antibody. Finally, he cites an experiment to suggest that the hemolysin-erythrocyte combination is not a chemical union. This result will later be known as the

Danysz or Bordet-Danysz phenomenon.[34] The addition of red cells in small aliquots absorbs the antibody more efficiently than adding the cells all at once. This should not occur in a chemical equilibrium union, says Bordet, but is typical of the variable adsorption of dyes by a piece of filter paper.

Bordet then summarizes those areas in which his data agree with Ehrlich, again failing each time to mention Ehrlich by name. He shows, using red-cell stromata (hemolyzed erythrocyte ghosts), that antibody is fixed, since the stroma can absorb it all from the antiserum. He shows that an "anti-hemolysin" *(sérum antihémolytique)* may be formed by repeated injections of guinea pig anti-rabbit blood (hemolytic serum) into new rabbits. This serum, when premixed with the hemolytic serum, appears to protect rabbit red cells from its hemolytic action. (Again, as discussed previously, it is not realized that the rabbit anti-guinea pig serum contains antibodies against all guinea pig serum proteins, thus fixing all available complement and rendering the red cells safe from hemolysis.) But Bordet reports a rather striking observation in this context; when he injects a large amount of the guinea pig anti-rabbit blood back into the rabbit, it is *immediately lethal.* He reports a picture of "disseminated hemorrhagic suffusions." The rapidity and pathologic changes described make it possible that this was one of the earliest observations of a form of systemic anaphylactic shock, such as would later be reported by Portier and Richet.[35] (There would, in any event, be a massive hemolytic crisis in the rabbit so treated.)

Bordet then proceeds to demonstrate that his anti-hemolysin serum also contains an anti-alexine (anti-complement), employing an experimental approach analogous to the one previously described. This also would have appeared logical, since the immunizing anti-erythrocyte serum also contains complement, and the resulting antiserum appears to inhibit the action of complement, just as it seems to inhibit the action of hemolytic antibody. But the results point to another conclusion; whereas there is no specificity in the action of complement (i.e., complements of many different species are all effective in mediating the hemolysis of rabbit cells), the "anti-complement" appears to be specific! Thus, rabbit "anti-guinea pig complement" will neutralize the complement activity of guinea pig serum, but not that of rabbit serum—again, the complement-fixing properties of the of anti-guinea pig serum proteins are not appreciated. It is interesting that Bordet mentions in passing[36] that the rabbit "anti-guinea pig complement" causes a precipitate when mixed either with the hemolytic or with normal guinea pig serum. Neither the nature of this precipitate nor its possible implications for the fixation of complement are mentioned, nor will they be until Bordet and Gengou[37] and Gengou[38] later show that *any* antigen–antibody interaction will fix complement.

Bordet then questions any priority of discovery that Ehrlich and Morgenroth may have claimed, still never mentioning them by name. He assigns the discovery of the specificity of lytic antibodies to Pfeiffer;[39] the demonstration of the passive transfer of cytolytic activity is credited to Fraenkel and Sobernheim;[40] the demonstration that these lytic reactions may be studied *in vitro* is assigned to Metchnikoff;[41] and a satisfactory theory of cytolysis he claims for himelf, "one that we advanced in 1895, and which our later investigations have been able to confirm entirely *without the addition of anything essential*" [my italics].

Bordet then passes in review the principal elements of his findings and conclusions, which he does not hesitate to call *la Théorie de Bordet*. But in a lengthy footnote he protests,

> We have observed with surprise that certain authors, especially in Germany, write a quite inexact history of these notions, sometimes attributing the study of these matters to authors who have only quite recently addressed these questions. In consequence, we will allow ourselves to cite verbatim certain passages from our communication of 1895 [note 12]. On pages 480 and 481 one reads. ... On page 499...

Thus, point by point, Bordet attempts to correct the record where he feels that his work has been slighted by others; clearly Ehrlich and Morgenroth are meant to be the culprits. He then discusses the theory advanced by Pfeiffer *(by name!)* to explain the lysis by antibody of cholera organisms, dealing much more gently with this latter investigator.

Ehrlich's Third Report: A Theory of Tolerance

The next communication on hemolysis by Ehrlich and Morgenroth appeared in May 1900.[42] It is a truly remarkable document, and forcefully illustrates the workings of a highly logical imagination. By this time Ehrlich would have become aware of the increasing interest in all sorts of destructive anti-cell antibodies, stimulated initially by the reports on anti-erythrocyte antibodies. He would have seen the reports on antispermatozoa by Landsteiner,[43] Metchnikoff,[44] and Metalnikoff;[45] of anti-ciliated epithelium by von Dungern;[46] and of anti-leukocyte antibodies by Besredka.[47] He also would have seen the provocative article by Metchnikoff on spermotoxic antibodies and their putative anti-antibodies.[48] In this report, Metchnikoff had injected guinea pig anti-rabbit spermatozoa serum into a rabbit and obtained a serum that inhibited the spermicidal action of the original antiserum. Just as Ehrlich had in an analogous experiment previously described, Metchnikoff interpreted this as the formation of of an anti-antibody that interacts with and neutralizes the anti-spermatozoa antibodies. Once again, a seemingly logical and reasonable interpretation led an investigator down what would prove to be a blind alley.

Having begun the report with mention of these anti-cell studies, and with the reminder that the side-chain theory holds that antibodies are cell receptors, Ehrlich and Morgenroth point out that everyone has worked with the injection of *foreign* cells. But such injections are unphysiological. Moreover, the formation of *auto*-antibodies should be theoretically possible since,

> If an animal organism, when injected with blood cells of foreign species, always produces a specific hemolysin for each of these species, it must surely be following a natural law; and it is improbable that this law ... should be suspended in the case of blood cells of the same individual. On the other hand, it is not to be denied that the formation of such hemolytic substances would appear dysteleological in the highest degree.[49]

But, they point out, the individual suffers the breakdown and absorption of its own cells and tissues in a variety of pathological conditions, from the action of toxins, hemorrhage, parenchymal atrophy, and so on. Why do these instances not lead to the development of autoantibodies and an antibody-mediated autodestruction? "It cannot be doubted that the organism seeks a way out of this difficulty by means of certain regulatory contrivances, the explanation of which would be of the highest interest." This, then, will be the object of the present studies.

They begin by injecting a goat with a mixture of the blood of three other goats, and test the resulting serum on the red cells of nine other goats. Six of them are strongly hemolyzed, two are hemolyzed only weakly, and one is entirely resistant, *as are the red cells of the immunized goat itself.* Three other goats are similarly immunized with the same mixture of goat blood; in each case, lysins for some but not all goats are obtained, and in no instance are the animal's own red cells affected. Interestingly, each of the four preparations differs in the set of animals whose erythrocytes it can hemolyze. (Here were the data that might have served for the description of blood groups, had they been analyzed from this direction. That same year, Karl Landsteiner would publish a similar analysis of human blood groups,[50] for which he would receive the Nobel Prize in 1930.)

It was clear to the authors that the species relationship of donor antigen and recipient antibody-producer are important. They therefore define the three different antibodies that might be formed: *heterolysins,* resulting from the response to antigens from a foreign species; *isolysins,* against antigens from a member of the same species; and *autolysins,* if an animal should respond to its own native antigens. But since hemolytic iso-antibodies are so readily produced and interact with so many red cell types, why do they not act on the cells of the animal that produced them (i.e., function as auto-antibodies)? Since all toxins and hemolysins must fix to cell receptors in order to exert their destructive activity, two possibilities are offered: either the blood cells entirely lack this receptor for isolysins, or they have receptors that are blocked by the animal's own auto-antibodies. The latter suggestion must be discarded, for "it would be incomprehensible that the blood-cells were not lysed by the complement also circulating in the blood." From this conclusion and in keeping with the side-chain theory, it is an easy jump to the conclusion that an animal does not produce auto-antibodies because it lacks the side-chain receptors specific for those auto-antigens. This is further generalized: "In the development or non-development of antibodies we shall have an indication of the presence or absence of receptors."[51] (We see here a bit of circular reasoning that will lead to problems in the future.)

The authors now develop the conceptual scheme to its logical conclusion. They point out that every red cell possesses a large number of different side-chains with haptophore groups (in modern parlance, epitopes) on its surface. Considering only a single group, let us inject that red cell into a recipient. If the immunized animal has appropriate receptors, it will make a hemolytic antibody; if it has no such receptors, no antibody will be formed. But if antibody is formed, two further possibilities exist: if the recipient does not possess the same antigenic grouping on *its own* cells, then the antibody titer will rise uninteruptedly and function only as an isolysin and not as an autolysin. However, if the recipient should possess the same antigenic grouping on its own erythrocytes, then these antibodies might function as destructive autolysins, causing much damage. But this does not appear to occur. Either the lysin's target receptors are routinely absent or, more likely according to Ehrlich and Morgenroth, are present, but another process intervenes. This is the formation of an anti-autolysin, effectively neutralizing the autolysin itself.

How does this occur? Simply by the fact that the autolysin, in interacting with *its* specific receptor, finds both an antigen *and an antibody,* that is, an anti-antibody. This is because the side-chain theory requires that any molecule with a haptophore group that finds a specific receptor to attach to induces the liberation of that receptor as a circulating antibody. If the eliciting molecule is itself an antibody, then the response must be the formation of an anti-antibody, and thus the neutralization of the one by the other. Note also that by virtue of their interaction with the same site on the antibody, the combining sites on the antigen and the anti-antibody must be identical! *Here is Jerne's network theory of immunoregulation*[52] already prefigured some 70 years in advance.[53]

The authors close this paper by pointing out that they have not yet observed an instance of auto-antibody formation, but will continue the search "until a lucky coincidence leads us [to it]." Not doubting the existence of the phenomenon, they go on to discuss the general problem of auto-intoxication in humans, some of which may be due to the normal breakdown and absorption of a variety of cells in the body. "Only when the internal regulatory contrivances are no longer intact can great dangers arise."

THE LAST ROUND:
THE POWER OF PURE LOGIC

Ehrlich's Fourth Report

On Hemolysis

The paper[54] opens with a review of the Ehrlich side-chain view of the nature of hemolytic antibody and complement. This is accompanied by an illustrative cartoon (Fig. 7.2) of the type that Ehrlich introduced in his Croonian Lecture. The interbody (hemolytic antibody) is represented as a toxin, by comparison with the toxins of tetanus or diphtheria. Whereas the latter constitutes a single molecule with a cell receptor-binding group and a toxic moiety, the former has two binding groups—one for the cell and the other for (toxic/enzymatic) complement.

The authors then review their notions about complement and hemolytic antibody. They point out that a serum may contain many different antibodies specific for the red cells of different species. Thus, rabbit erythrocytes will absorb all anti-rabbit hemolytic antibody from a heated serum, while leaving behind a functional anti-guinea pig hemolysin. They even suggest that a hemolytic serum active on a

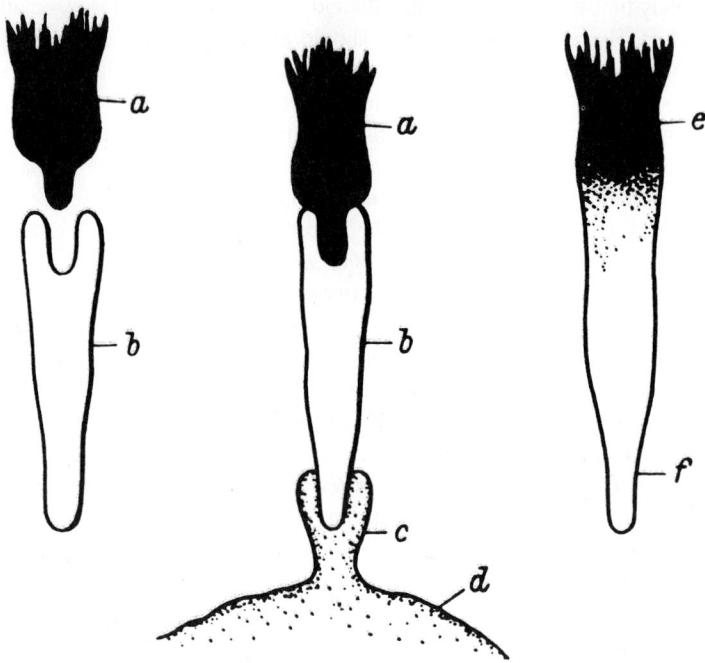

FIGURE 7.2   Ehrlich's demonstration of the similarity between the structure of the hemolytic antibody-complement complex and the structure of diphtheria or tetanus toxin. a = complement; b = hemolytic antibody; c = the erythrocyte receptor; d = the red cell; e = the toxophore group on the toxin; and f = the combining site on the toxin. (After Ehrlich, note 54.)

given red cell may consist of a mixture of different antibodies, presumably based on differences in their affinity for different complements—this harks back to the Ehrlich's diphtheria antitoxin studies described in Chapter 5. Further, they insist again that there is a multiplicity of different complements, each different hemolysin bearing a receptor for its own specific effector molecule.

In countering Buchner's objections[55] to the existence of a multiplicity of complements they say in words that Bordet might have used, "we must emphasize that our conclusions are not the result of speculation, but simply the necessary consequences of observations which are not to be harmonized with the assumption of a single simple alexin."[56] It is of further interest that Ehrlich, ever conscious of the clinical correlates of his work, notes that a profound complementopenia accompanies systemic phosphorus poisoning.

On Anti-Complements

The authors then review their earlier findings that the injection of complement-rich sera from one species into another will result in the formation of

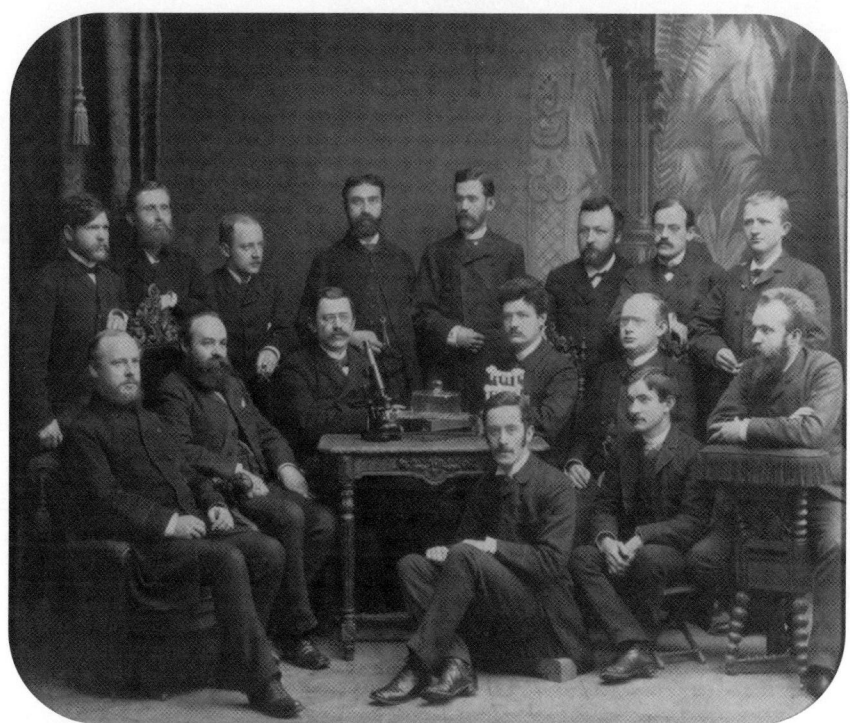

PLATE 1 Julius Cohnheim's pathology group, Breslau, in the summer of 1877. Cohnheim is standing fourth from left. On his left is the young medical student Paul Ehrlich. Seated at far left is visiting American pathologist William Welch; seated next to him is Ehrlich's cousin Carl Weigert. Seated at the far right is visiting Danish microbiologist Carl Julius Salomonsen. (Courtesy Johns Hopkins Medical Archives.)

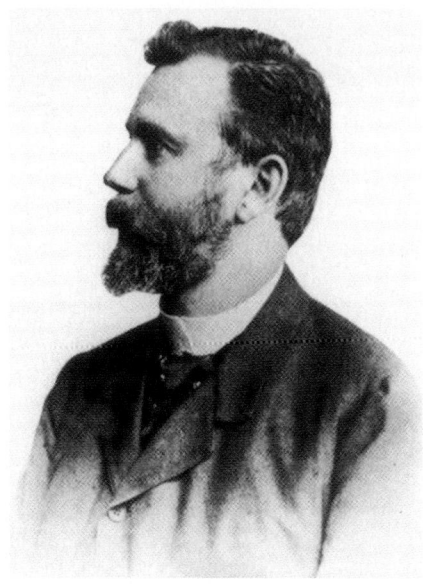

PLATE 2   Paul Ehrlich during his Berlin days, about 1890.

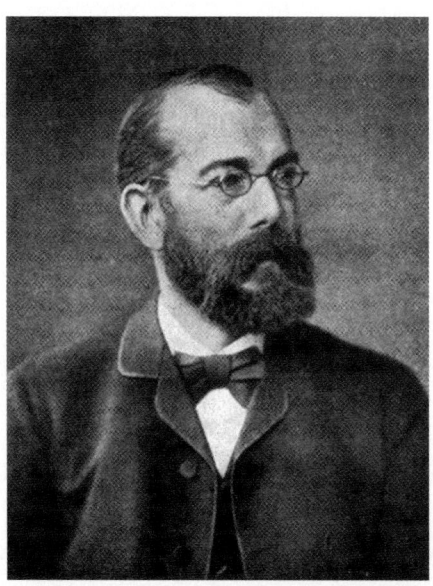

PLATE 3   Robert Koch (Courtesy, National Library of Medicine.)

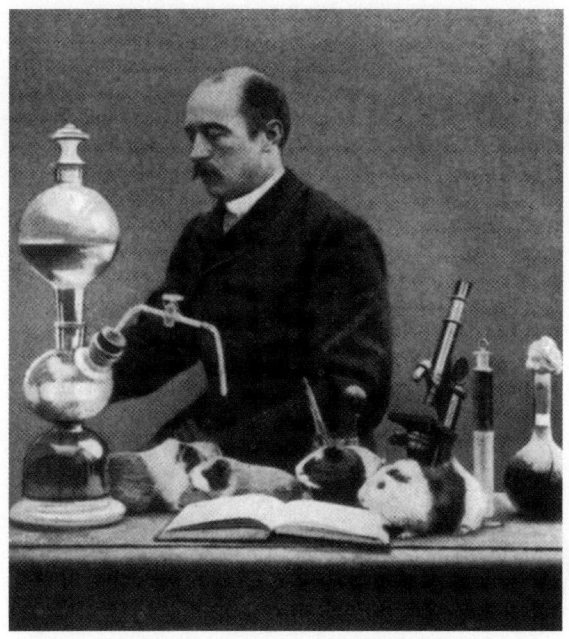

PLATE 4   Emil Behring (Courtesy National Library of Medicine.)

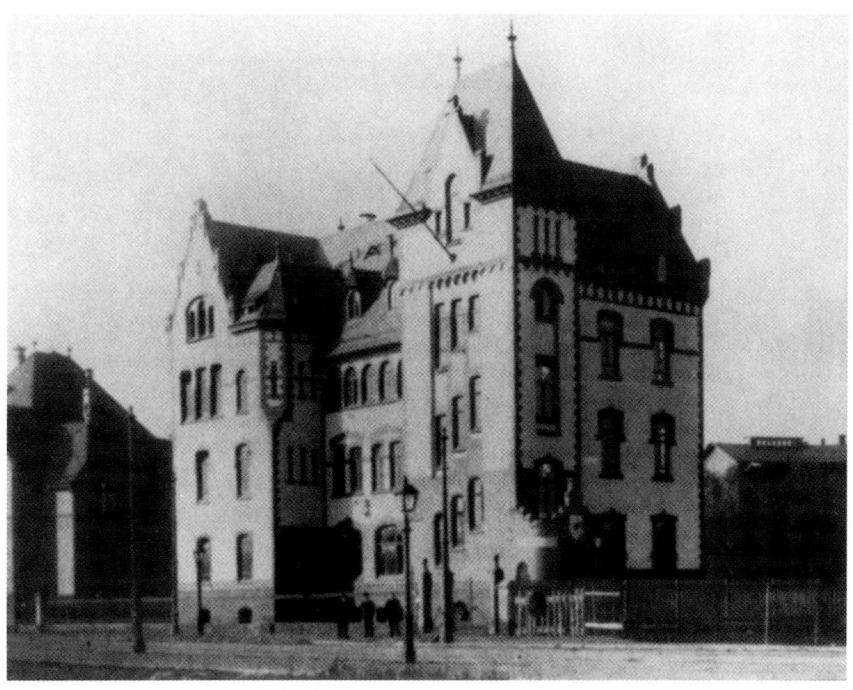

PLATE 5   The Royal Institute for Experimental Therapy, Frankfurt am Main, 1900.

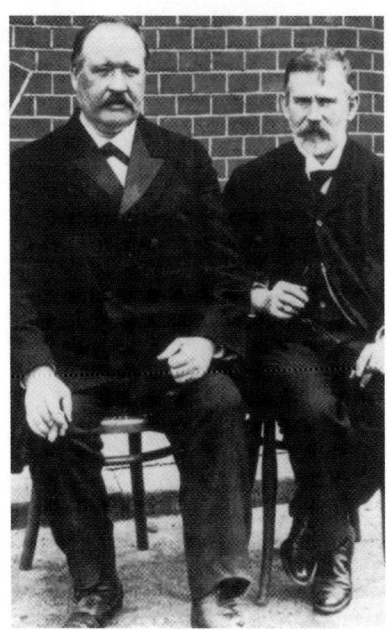

PLATE 6   Ehrlich and Svante Arrhenius, 1903.

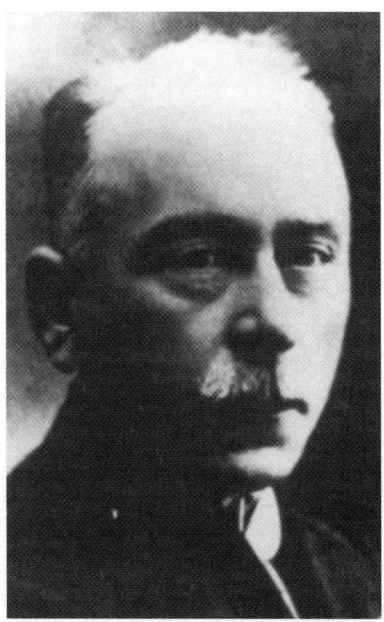

PLATE 7   Jules Bordet. (Courtesy Institut Pasteur, Paris.)

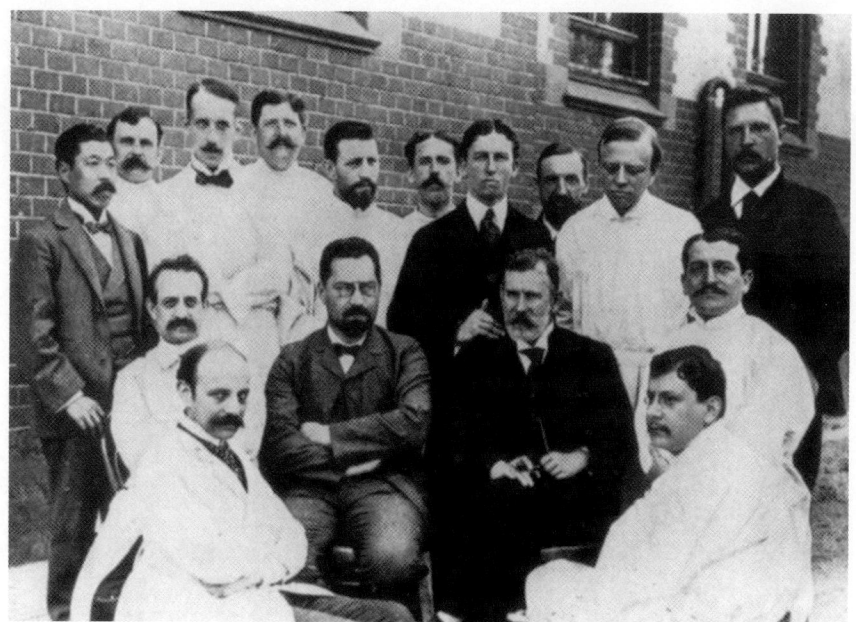

PLATE 8   Ehrlich and associates, about 1903. Morgenroth is seated on Ehrlich's right; Shiga is standing on the far left.

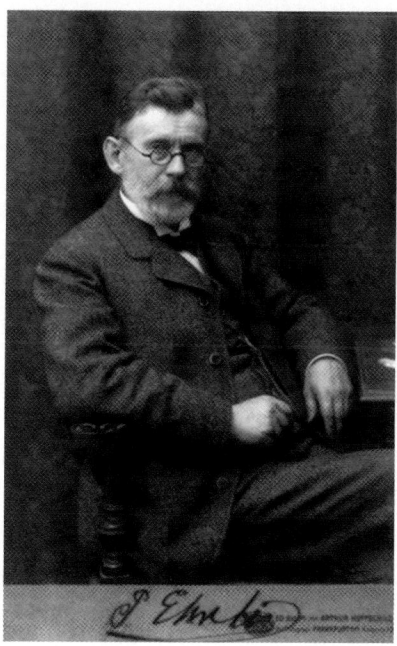

PLATE 9   Ehrlich at age 50.

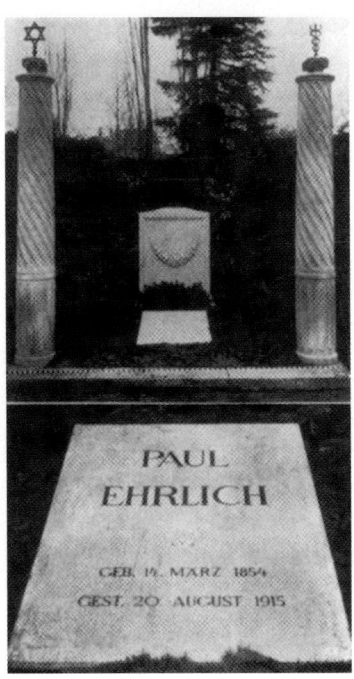

PLATE 10 Ehrlich's gravesite, Frankfurt am Main. (Above) The site is marked by columns with the Star of David and the Caduceus. (Below) An enlargement of the stone marker.

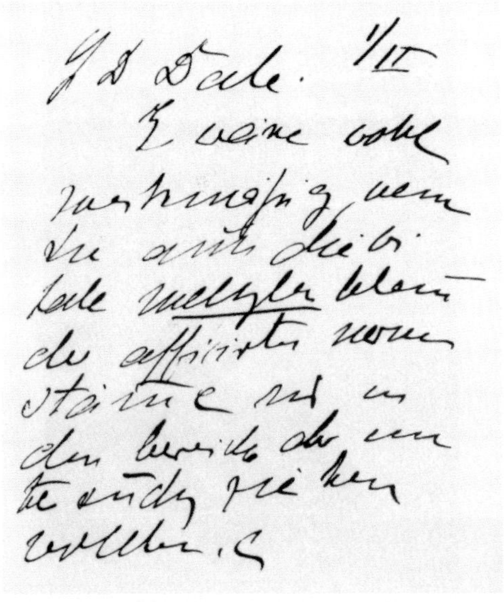

PLATE 11 One of Ehrlich's famous almost-illegible notes *(Blöke)*, addressed to Henry Dale. "It would perhaps be appropriate if you would apply the vital [stain] methylene blue to the affected nerve stem in your investigation."

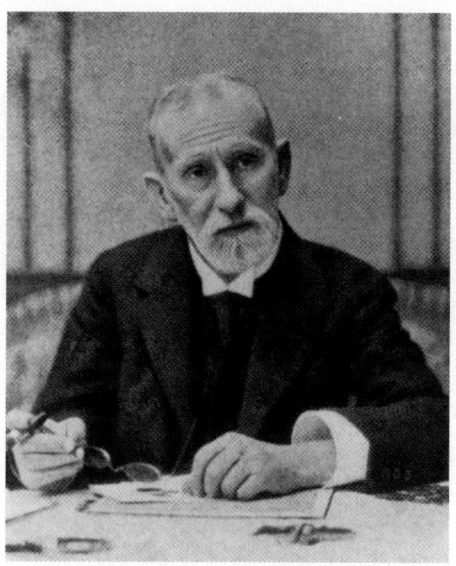

PLATE 12   Ehrlich's last portrait, taken shortly before his death.

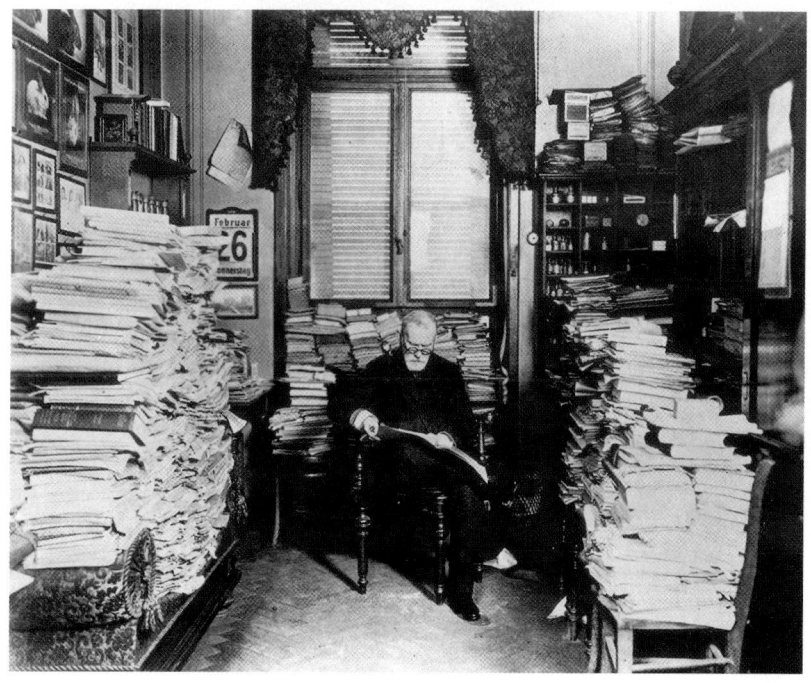

PLATE 13   Ehrlich's crowded office at his Frankfurt Institute, February 26, 1914.

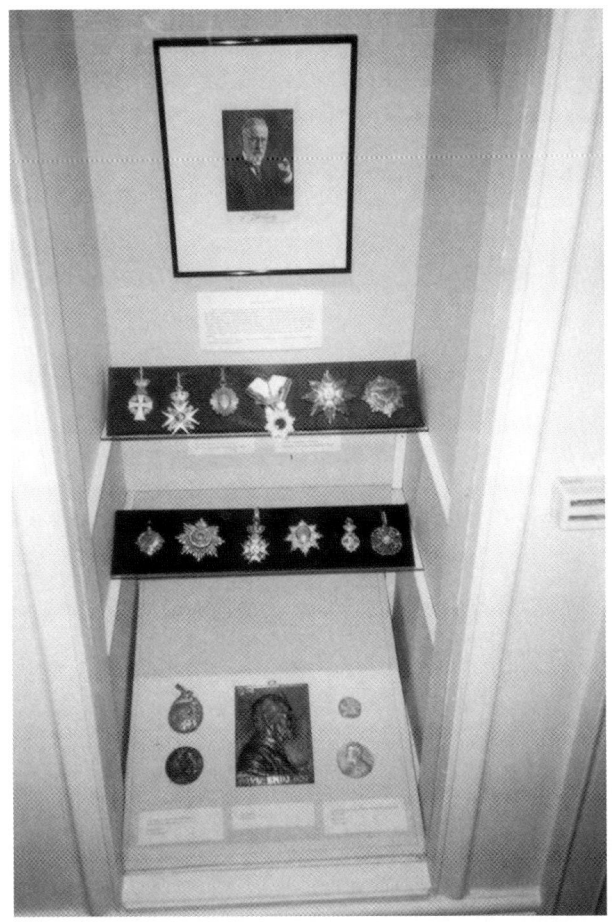

PLATE 14   Ehrlich's medals, on display at the Rockefeller Archives Center, Sleepy Hollow, New York. (With permission.)

"anti-complements." As noted previously, such an antiserum will neutralize the complement activity of the target serum when they are mixed, and logic demands that the explanation lay in the development of an anti-complement. But complement has two active groupings according to the side-chain theory: a haptophore to mediate its attachment to the antibody, and a toxophore to effect hemolysis. Therefore the anti-complement could be directed at one or both of these groupings.

The logic of the design of the experiment to clarify the nature of the anti-complement was impeccable. If the anti-complement is directed against the toxic end, then the combining end would be free to attach to the antibody, thus "clogging" all of these sites and rendering them inaccessible to fresh active complement. On the other hand, if the antibody is directed against the combining site on the complement, adding it to sensitized cells would have no effect on the complement-fixing site on the hemolytic antibody, and fresh complement would mediate hemolysis. The results were clear. Red cells were sensitized with heated antiserum and then washed. They were then treated with a mixture of a complement-rich serum and its respective "anti-complement" and washed again. The addition of a fresh source of complement resulted in rapid lysis of the target erythrocytes. As the authors conclude, *"the anticomplement acts by fitting into the haptophore group of the complement and side-tracking this group"* [their italics].

The remainder of the paper is devoted to an attack on Bordet's theory and his interpretation of his data. Bordet had argued the *unitarian* thesis of complement from the qualitative observations that the complements of many different species can mediate the hemolysis of rabbit red cells treated with guinea pig anti-rabbit hemolytic serum. Ehrlich and Morgenroth object, and call upon quantitative data that show that the complements of some species act much more efficiently than do those of other species, and thus must not only differ but be composed of mixtures of many different complement types. Moreover, they posit the existence of multiple antibodies specific for the given target erythrocyte, often present in differing ratios, and each utilizing its own specific complement. In this case, as with the toxin spectra described in Chapter 5, *any* result can be explained by the choice of appropriate ratios of the several components active in the process. Indeed, the authors hint that they may have understated the complexity of the situation, and that "thorough, though to be sure arduous, studies will show a multiplicity heretofore unexpected. ... For the present, however, this duality of the immune-body should suffice to refute the objections made by Bordet from the unitarian standpoint."[57]

In his concluding remarks to the 1906 English edition of his *Collected Studies*,[58] Ehrlich would recognize the many observations showing that the injection of a serum results in the formation of multiple antibodies, each potentially capable of fixing complement. Although insisting that these be considered amboceptors also, he concedes that, "This being the case, the demonstration of anticomplements by immunization becomes extremely difficult."

Ehrlich's Fifth Report

The paper, published in March 1901,[59] opens with the declaration that the side-chain theory, developed in the context of toxins and antitoxins, has been thoroughly vindicated. If indeed it has any general biological applicability beyond toxins, then it should also be able to explain the immune response to tissue cells and bacteria. This is why the authors have studied immune hemolysis as a critical test of the theory, a phenomenon whose discovery they now unequivocally credit to Jules Bordet for the very first time. But they point out that new systems may require minor adjustments to existing theories, just as hemolysis has required a modification of the side-chain theory of antitoxins. In no way should this be considered a weakness of a valid theory, but it will instead result in a deeper understanding of the subject. They illustrate this point by reference to the famous theory of solutions of van't Hoff, which holds that osmotic pressure depends on the number of particles in a solution. When the theory was threatened by the aberrant osmotic results observed with salt solutions, Arrhenius's concept of electrolytic dissociation not only explained the anomaly but reinforced the original theory.

This analogy provided a useful segue to a discussion of the chemical basis of the combinations of antibody with cell and of antibody with complement. The analogy was made between hemolytic antibody and a chemical with two active groups (such as a diazo group at one end and an aldehyde at the other), able to "connect" two reactive substances to one another across this bridge. For the first time, they would coin the term "amboceptor" to describe this two-headed (or rather, two-grasping-handed) physiological substance.

The Bordet–Danysz Paradox

The authors next take up the accusation made by Bordet that the combination of antibody with erythrocyte cannot be a chemical union, but must rather be like the adsorption of dyes by filter paper. Bordet had noted that if the hemolytic dose of an antibody is established for a given quantity of red cells, then it is found that all of the antibody is taken up when only half that quantity of cells is added, leaving nothing to mediate hemolysis on addition of the second aliquot. For Ehrlich, this presented no problem of interpretation. He pointed out that the erythrocyte might contain many more receptor sites for antibody than are needed to mediate hemolysis. Given his ideas on the tight, essentially irreversible chemical binding of antibody haptophore group to the cell receptor, a cell with twice the minimum number of receptors may bind two hemolytic doses of antibody before any additional would be found free in the supernatant. Indeed, they show experimentally that the total number of binding sites may vary from one antibody-red cell combination to another, sometimes achieving a value of 100 times the number needed for hemolysis. The side-chain theory is preserved!

The picture is made clear with a chemical analogy. Naphthalene diamine possesses two sites able to combine with a diazo compound. One aliquot of diazo compound is sufficient to form a colored product (the mono-azo compound), but addition of double that amount will combine totally (the di-substituted product), leaving no reagent free in solution.

Now Ehrlich brings to bear his most potent argument against Bordet's theory of dye-like adsorption—specificity. He points out that charcoal and other surface-active substances can attract thousands of different substances of the most varied type. Further, any given dye may stain a large number of different substances. Where in the absorption of dyes, asks Ehrlich, is the specificity so characteristic of immunological interactions? A rabbit anti-guinea pig hemolysin reacts only with guinea pig erythrocytes. Where there is a cross-reaction that might suggest a breakdown of specificity, as when a goat anti-goat isolysin is found to act on sheep red cells, it can be shown by specific absorption that the two species have receptors in common.

Complementoids

There now appeared one of those typical Ehrlichean conceptual leaps, in which the inner logic of a phenomenon seems to demand the step-by-step elaboration of an earlier theory. We saw previously (Fig. 7.2) that complement was viewed as a bipolar molecule, one end the toxic moiety and the other the binding site, by analogy with tetanus and diphtheria toxins. But if the bacterial toxins can be converted into *toxoids,* now innocuous but still capable of eliciting antitoxic antibody, why not the hemolytic ones? Perhaps the inactivation of complement by heating serves only to diminish the toxicity of the hemolytic "zymotoxic" end, turning it into a complementoid.

The test of this hypothesis was easy. Heat-inactivated goat complement was injected into various species, and in each instance an antiserum was formed that specifically inhibited the activity of fresh goat complement. But the antisera to heat-inactivated complements seemed to function the same as that against fresh, active complements. Thus, they could conclude that, "according to our view that it is the haptophore group which causes the immunity reaction, it follows that *inactivation of the complement has destroyed only the zymotoxic group, leaving the haptophore group intact*" [their italics].[60] However, if the "complementoid" has an intact binding site, then heat-inactivated complement should compete with fresh complement for binding to the antibody and thus inhibit its action. Since it appears not to do this, logic requires that, *"in the change to complementoid, the haptophore group of the complement suffers a diminution of its affinity for the complementophile group of the immune-body"* [their italics]. They assume that in this instance, the two active sites on the molecule are close enough to one another so that altering the one will exert an effect on the other. Similar experiments seeming to support the existence of complementoids were later published by Ehrlich and Sachs.[61]

Auto-Anticomplements and Horror Autotoxicus

Ehrlich and Morgenroth recall that in their third communication on hemolysins, they discussed the implications of the formation of cytotoxic antibodies against self. They pointed out that there must exist "certain contrivances by means of which the immunity reaction, so easily produced by all kinds of cells, is prevented from acting against the organism's own elements and so giving rise to autotoxins." They term this general physiological process *Horror Autotoxicus,* or the "fear" of self-intoxication. In a footnote, they point out that Metalnikoff's observation of anti-spermatozoal antibodies[62] does not contradict this principle; the antibody attaches but the spermatozoa survive, and thus, "an autotoxin within our meaning, *one that destroys the cells of the organism that formed it,* does not exist" [italics in the original].

Now, in their study of complements and anticomplements, they believe that they have observed another manifestation of this phenomenon. They found that about 1 week after the injection of large amounts of goat serum into rabbits (with the object of producing rabbit anti-goat complement), the rabbit's own complement seemed to disappear, not to return until some weeks later. Indeed, this complement-free serum even neutralized the complement present in fresh rabbit serum. The conclusion seems inescapable—since the rabbit does not spontaneously form antibodies against its own complement, the goat complements must share cross-reacting constituents with the rabbit's own complements, so that the anti-goat complement formed by the rabbit must be considered an *auto-anti-complement.* (Here is the prediction, long forgotten, that would be rediscovered and confirmed a half-century later by researchers studying the "breaking" of tolerance by cross-reacting antigens.) Further, the clinical consequences of such a complement deficiency are mentioned; they quote preliminary findings by Neisser and Wechsberg to the effect that such animals suffer a decreased resistance to certain infections, testimony to the important function of complement.

Once again, the logic is impeccable, given the demands of Ehrlich's side-chain theory and the contemporary view of the nature of the reagents and methods employed. A fresh, complement-rich serum was viewed as complement alone; if it were derived from an immunized animal, then it might be considered to possess two components, antibody and complement. If it were employed to immunize an animal, then the resulting antibodies could only be specific for the presumed contents of the serum. Again, the doses employed for immunization were large by later standards; to produce hemolytic antisera, 10 cc or more *of whole blood* might be used, and similar volumes of serum to produce "anti-antibodies" or "anti-complements." The presence of untold numbers of other immunogenic proteins in these inocula was not appreciated.

The full explanation of the phenomenon of complement depletion following the administration of massive doses of serum would appear in 1910, although it would not be fully appreciated at the time. It will be recalled that Behring's treatment of diphtheria and tetanus involved the administration of large doses of horse antitoxic serum; in many instances, while the toxic disease was cured, a curious side reaction would occur beginning a week or so later. This was called *serum sickness.* Its pathogenesis would be explained by Clemens Baron von Pirquet, in a

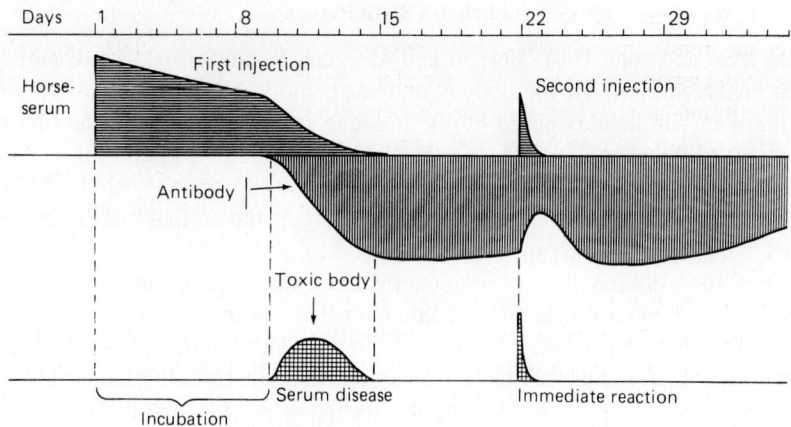

FIGURE 7.3   von Pirquet's concept of the steps in the development of serum sickness. (After Pirquet, *Allergy,* note 63.)

remarkable demonstration of insight, in a book entitled *Allergy.*[63] The story is worth retelling here, since it illustrates how some distant connections may be made in a field, while other closer connections may be missed.

By 1910, the following observations had been made:

1. The mixture of antibody with antigens would form a visible precipitate.[64]
2. Serum contains much protein, and antibodies may be formed against serum protein antigens.[65]
3. The interaction of antibody with antigen may cause systemic anaphylaxis[66] or local hemmorhagic necrosis.[67]
4. Any antigen-antibody combination can fix complement.[68]

Now comes Pirquet the pediatrician, long interested in the clinical consequences of serum sickness that he had identified some years earlier, in collaboration with Bela Schick.[69] Pirquet proposed a pathogenesis of serum sickness that was made perfectly clear in a single diagram in his book—we reproduce it here in Figure 7.3. Note how well it illustrates the steps in the immune response that would be the subject of study of a later generation of immunologists. An injection of serum protein is made, which only slowly leaves the circulation over the next week or so. Then, suddenly, with the onset of antibody formation, the antigen disappears more rapidly in what would later be termed the phase of immune elimination. At the same time, a "toxic body" is formed, presumably the antigen–antibody complex precipitin formed *in vivo;* this is the material responsible for the clinical manifestations of the disease. Antibody formation continues, so that a repeated injection of the same serum will result in an immediate reaction, due to the formation of new immune complexes.

Ehrlich's Sixth Report

In May and June 1901, Ehrlich and Morgenroth published the two parts of their final contribution to the study of immune hemolysis.[70] It opens with a review of the many difficulties posed by the immune response in general, and by the study of cytotoxic antibodies in particular. They mention the curious observation that the usual antibody response in frogs is suppressed when they are kept in the cold.[71] This is ascribed, reasonably, to a slowing of the normal metabolic functions in this cold-blooded species.

They also discuss the observation by most investigators that an antibody response is often undetectable in certain animals or in certain species. This, they hold, can only be due to one of two causes, in the context of the side-chain theory: either the animal's cells lack the necessary receptors that would become antibodies when cast off from the cell, or the receptors are too tightly bound to be released. They call these *sessile receptors,* reminiscent of the "sessile" antibodies that would be postulated three to four decades later to explain delayed hypersensitivity reactions.

On the Multiplicity of Antibodies

The authors report that the immunization of rabbits with ox red cells results in a hemlytic serum that acts on goat erythrocytes as well. This is true of every rabbit tried, but the ratio of anti-ox to anti-goat titers differs from 1.5:1 to 17:1, showing a marked variation among individuals. In each instance, substantially all of the anti-ox and anti-goat activity can be absorbed from the serum using ox cells, but absorption with goat cells leaves the anti-ox hemolytic activity unaffected. When the reverse experiment is performed, immunizing several rabbits with goat red cells, the ratio of anti-goat to anti-ox titers varies from 2.4:1 to 33:1. Now absorption with goat erythrocytes removes almost all activity against both cell types, whereas absorption with ox cells leaves the anti-goat activity undiminished. Here again is one of the early examples of the use of differential absorption of cross-reacting antisera.[72]

The explanation offered for this apparent interspecies cross-reaction lies in the sharing of antigenic sites on the two red cell types. This is because Ehrlich's theory does not allow for multiple antibodies specific for the *same* antigenic site. This concept is represented pictorially in Figure 7.4, where each cell contains a target site unique to that species as well as a different site shared between species. This result reinforces Ehrlich's view that the surface of all cells must contain a large variety of antigenic sites (as well as, we might note, receptor sites that can be shed as circulating antibodies). The further consequence of this is that each antiserum must consist of *"several, perhaps a host of, immune-bodies"* [their italics, note 70, p. 285]. This conclusion appears to be confirmed by the earlier observation that a goat might produce a variety of anti-goat isolysins. Here is a subtle correction to an earlier view; no longer is the entire antiserum specific; rather, it is composed of a mixture of many individually specific antibodies.

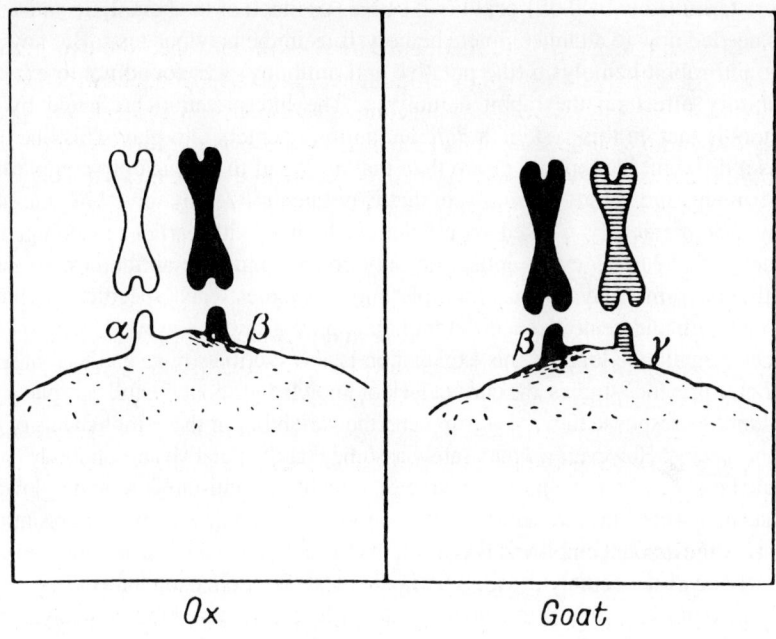

FIGURE 7.4 Ehrlich's demonstration of the hemolytic cross-reaction between ox and goat red cells. Some antigenic receptors are shared (β), whereas others are unique to the species (α, γ). (After Ehrlich and Morgenroth, note 70.)

Anti-Antibodies

Ehrlich and Morgenroth next report a complex series of experiments designed to confirm the existence and action of anti-antibodies specific for the combining sites (cytophilic groups) on the hemolytic antibodies. They have obtained a very high-titer rabbit anti-ox hemolytic serum and used it to immunize a goat. (Note that, following a common practice, they have injected the goat with as much as 120 cc (!) of the whole rabbit serum over a period of 2 months.) They then mix 0.5 cc of this "anti-antibody" with increasing amounts of the rabbit hemolytic serum (of which 0.001 cc constitutes a hemolytic unit). To this mixture is then added a standard suspension of ox red cells, the mixture incubated, centrifuged, and the sedimented red cells resuspended and then exposed to the action of excess guinea pig complement. The tests were controlled using normal goat serum in place of the goat anti-rabbit serum. It was found that the goat anti-rabbit serum would inhibit up to 17.5 hemolytic units of the rabbit anti-ox hemolysin.

The same experiment was run using goat complement in place of the guinea pig complement previously employed. In this system, the rabbit anti-ox hemolytic unit was determined to be 0.051 cc; thus, 51 times as much of the hemolytic antiserum was needed now to attain complete hemolysis as in the previous tests. But now the goat anti-rabbit hemolysin (the putative anti-antibody) was found not to exert an inhibitory effect on the rabbit hemolysin. The interpretation presented by the authors is that, in this system, a *different* antibody enters into play. This one contains a different haptophore group than that acting in the guinea pig complement experiment, and is thus a hemolysin that is not neutralized by the rabbit anti-antibody that previously worked so efficiently. In line with earlier reasoning, it is assumed that just as every antiserum may contain multiple antibodies, so every "anti-antiserum" may contain multiple anti-antibodies, each specifically able to interact with and neutralize a different haptophore group.

Once again, the logic of this explanation is above criticism, given the context of Ehrlich's previous studies, the current lack of knowledge about the full complexity of the immune response to whole serum, and the variability of the complements of different species. However, we may safely assume that the putative anti-antibody (what would be called later an anti-idiotype) was in reality an anti-rabbit immunoglobulin. As such, it would indeed neutralize the action of the rabbit anti-ox hemolysin; presumably the amount employed was adequate to neutralize all of the immunoglobulin in 0.017 cc of the hemolytic serum in the first test. But goat complement is so much less efficient than guinea pig complement that 51 times more rabbit hemolysin was required to furnish a hemolytic unit, following the now well-understood reciprocal relationship between hemolytic antibody and complement.[73] With so much rabbit serum present, the goat anti-rabbit serum could not have neutralized all the rabbit immunoglobulin in the test; unneutralized hemolysin would have remained active, and thus the "anti-antibody" would have appeared ineffective in this system. This supposition appears to be confirmed by the fact that the authors found that their goat anti-rabbit hemolytic serum (the anti-antibody) was essentially ineffective in neutralizing the anti-ox hemolysins formed in other species. Again, they assumed, reasonably, that this was due to the formation of hemolysins containing non-crossreactive haptophore groups, but it appears in retrospect to be due to the non-crossreactivity of the immunoglobulins of these different species.

The Multiplicity of Complements

The authors then present further experimental support for their view that there are many different complements—at least one for each of the different hemolytic antibodies they have observed. They extend the observation that the complements of different species affect the amount of rabbit anti-ox erythrocytes required to hemolyze ox cells. As we saw, many times more antibody is required in the presence of goat complement than is needed for guinea pig complement, and the values for such complements as rabbit, rat, goose, and chicken fall in-between. The explanation again is that the rabbit antibody is a mixture of many types, each requiring its own specific complement. The antibody mixture would thus be richer in antibodies specific for guinea pig complement than for other complements, and therefore the titer found with this complement would be higher.

They then compare their rabbit anti-ox erythrocyte serum with goose anti-ox erythrocyte serum, using the complements of different species to mediate the hemolytic reaction. The order of efficacies in these two systems is roughly comparable, but they wonder at the fact that goose and chicken complements work better in the rabbit antibody system than does horse complement, and pigeon complement seems not to be able to participate at all. They point out that this argues against the supposition that the zoological closeness of species should manifest itself in the similarity of action of such constituents as their complements, and thus against Bordet's unitarian theory of complement action. Once again, the explanation proferred is the existence of multiple complements, each acting only with its respective specific antibody.

Finally, the authors discuss the clinical implications of the existence of multiple antibodies and multiple complements. To best utilize all the complements present in a patient in the immunological fight against bacterial infection, it is advised that any passive antibody administered be derived from a mixture of different donors and even from different species.

Bordet Responds

In May 1901, Bordet repeated his arguments against Ehrlich's theory of the chemical interaction of amboceptors and complement, arguing once again for the theory of "sensitization."[74] Whereas this merely represented a restatement of positions in respect of antibody, a new observation was advanced against Ehrlich's contention that there exists a multiplicity of complements. Bordet shows that *all* the complement may be removed from a serum by an antibody-cell interaction, thus depriving other antibody-cell systems of its collaboration in lysis. Here is proof, says Bordet, that there is only a single complement.

This challenge to his theory was met by Ehrlich in a paper coauthored with Marshall, a Rockefeller Institute Fellow studying with Ehrlich in Frankfurt.[75] They argued that indeed each serum contains a multiplicity of complements. Therefore, if a given amboceptor were to fix many complements, it must be because that amboceptor contains receptor sites for each of them. They picture this structure in the now-familiar style adopted by Ehrlich, as illustrated in Figure 7.5. The amboceptor now possesses many different complementophilic sites, each specific for its respective complement—some were called "dominant" complements and others "nondominant." This is typical Ehrlich, building one *ad hoc* structure on another, as he had done with toxins to explain their neutralization spectra and with antibodies to explain the shift from simple antitoxins to the more complicated hemolysins.

SUMMARY

The stimulus provided by Jules Bordet's brief report on immune hemolysis elicited a burst of activity by Paul Ehrlich and his associates. The series of chal-

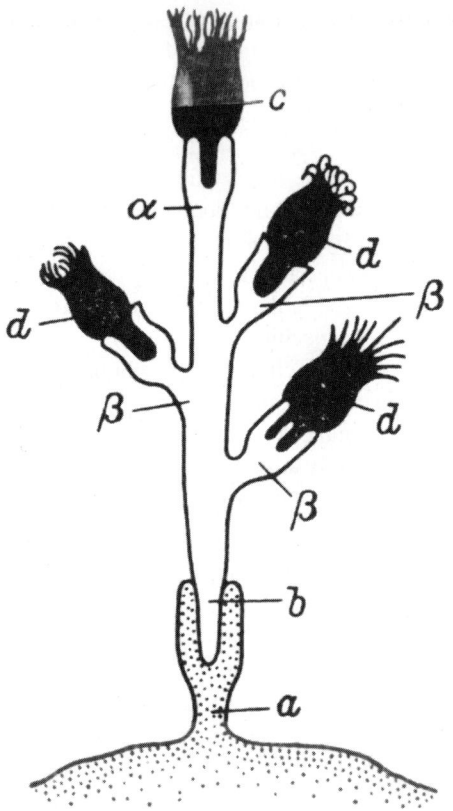

FIGURE 7.5 Ehrlich's explanation of why *any* immune complex could fix substantially all the complement in a serum. If the complement-antibody bond is specific, then each antibody must possess multiple binding sites, for both the "dominant" complement (c) and for all of the "non-dominant" ones (d). (After Ehrlich and Marshall, note 75.)

lenges, rebuttals, and counterchallenges that flew between the two laboratories resulted in a significant leap forward for immunology, both in the data obtained and in the new scientists attracted to this interesting and increasingly important field. Here is one of the best examples that differences of opinion and interpretation and unabashed challenge may be more productive of progress than quiet agreement among investigators.[76]

If anyone at the turn of the century would rush to the defense of his ideas, it was Paul Ehrlich. He combined a love of theory with elegance as an experimenter, and acted throughout as if his side-chain theory had been proved beyond doubt. Therefore its extension to immune hemolysis must be valid in all its aspects. Bordet, on the other hand, professed to be disinterested in theory and trusting only in facts. He insisted that the ideas that he put forward were not even worthy to be called theories. As he would later say,

> My single desire has been to show that it is not I myself who have created or even chosen my ideas; they have rather been forced upon me by facts, by the logical induction which, so to speak, is the inevitable result of experimentation, and by the immediate deductions from it. I have limited myself to being an experimenter and very little of a theorist, and the accuracy of the opinions which I have defended is, I think, guaranteed by this fact.[77]

But this statement would appear to be somewhat disingenuous. Bordet's introduction of physical adsorption, of colloidal properties of the components, and of the implications about mechanism implied by his *substance sensibilisatrice* were, if less detailed than Ehrlich's ideas, surely no less conceptual.[78] Indeed, the first sentence of the quote could have been uttered by Ehrlich himself, who was fully convinced that it was "the facts" that had stipulated his theories. Ehrlich, however, would not have been as modest as Bordet was in the second sentence of the quote; he would probably have insisted that the facts had to be organized and interpreted by a keen theoretical mind (such as he possessed).

Over the period of the next decade, the conceptual dispute between Ehrlich and Bordet slowly softened and declined; the various alarums and excursions published in the journals by the two protagonists and then by their followers became rarer as the years passed. In the end, as is so often true in science, the views of both sides would prove partially correct and partially in error. Ehrlich's concept of the stereochemical basis of antibody specificity (the haptophore group) would be validated, and his nomenclature (*Antikörper* and *Komplement*) would survive. But the idea of a "complementophile" group on hemolytic antibody would disappear. For his part, Bordet's notion of the "sensitization" of the red cell by antibody to permit the fixation of complement, and of the existence of but a single complement,[79] would be confirmed.

Whereas Ehrlich shifted his interests to experimental tumor research and chemotherapy (see Chapter 8) in the early years of the new century, Bordet continued to concentrate on immunology during the remainder of his scientific life. They both would eventually win the Nobel Prize for their immunology, Ehrlich sharing his with Elie Metchnikoff in 1908 and Bordet, finally, in 1919. Ehrlich died in 1915, and thus was spared the further modifications of his concepts that later data would have demanded. Bordet, however (who lived until 1961 at age 91), utilized the leisure enforced by World War I to write his magnum opus, *L'Immunité dans les Maladies Infectieuses* in 1919,[80] summarizing the field as it was then appreciated. In it, he treats Ehrlich's theories more gently than before, especially those that emphasize the chemical nature of immunological specificity. But the earlier battles are not completely forgotten; Bordet can still write,

> My predilection for realities has not been able to prevent me from briefly considering hypotheses, even reckless ones; they have left too profound an impression on many studies to be passed over in silence. One knows the luxurience with which they have been developed on the fertile terrain of immunology, where so much of the unknown still

stimulates the imagination and (it must be added) invites audaciously synthetic concepts from those schools anxious to affirm their superiority by inspired suppositions. Thus, general hypotheses crop up with dominating and conquering pretensions that wish in a single step to embrace an entire scientific territory and annex it thenceforth; thus are constructed tyrranical systems which are angered by facts which are difficult to incorporate and which are defended with all the prejudice that an amour-propre mixed with chauvinism so readily inspires.[81]

Thus, over the years, the dispute about the nature of the interaction between erythrocyte, hemolytic/hemagglutinating antibody, and complement slowly lost its polemical tones, without the declaration of a "winner" on either side. What remained, however, was a set of methodologies that contributed significantly to immunology and its allied sciences: the practical fields of diagnostic serology and immunohematology; the elucidation of the components of complement, perhaps the founding paradigm of the field of immunopharmacology; and the application of hemolytic plaque assays to study single cell responses and the cellular dynamics of the immune response.

NOTES AND REFERENCES

1. Bordet, J., *Ann. Inst. Pasteur* 12:688, 1898; English transl., F.P. Gay, ed., *Studies in Immunity*, New York, Wiley, 1909, pp. 134–141, (henceforth *Bordet Studies*).
2. Belfanti, S., and Carbone, T., *G.R. Acad. Torino* 46:321, 1898.
3. Bordet, J. and and Gengou, O., *Ann. Inst. Pasteur* 15:290, 1901; *Bordet Studies*, pp. 217–227.
4. Wassermann, A., Neisser, C., and Schucht, A., *Z. Hygiene* 55:451, 1906.
5. Some of the important consequences of Bordet's discovery of immune hemolysis are discussed in greater detail by Silverstein, A.M., *J. Hist. Biol.* 27:437, 1994.
6. Human blood groups were discoverd by Landsteiner, K., *Zentralbl. Bakteriol.* 27:357, 1900.
7. See. e.g., Lattes, L., *Die Individualität des Blutes*, Berlin, Springer, 1925, and Hirszfeld, L., *Ergeb. Hyg. Bakteriol.* 8:367, 1926.
8. Donath, J. and Landsteiner, K., *Münch. med. Wochenschr.* 51:1590, 1904.
9. Jerne, N.K. and Nordin, A.A., *Science* 140:405, 1963.
10. Pfeiffer, R., *Z. Hygiene* 18:1, 1894.
11. Metchnikoff, E., *Ann. Inst. Pasteur* 9:433, 1895.
12. Bordet, J., *Ann. Inst. Pasteur* 9:462, 1895; *Bordet Studies* pp. 56–80.
13. Buchner, H., *Zentralbl. Bakteriol.* 6:561, 1889.
14. Bordet, note 1, p. 695.
15. Ehrlich P. and Morgenroth, J., *Berlin klin. Wochenschr.*, 36:6–9, 1899; English transl. *Collected Papers of Paul Ehrlich*, London, Pergamon, 1956–1960, vol. II, pp. 143–149; henceforth, *Collected Papers*.
16. Zinsser, H., *J. Immunol.* 6:289, 1921.
17. Ehrlich and Morgenroth, *Collected Papers*, vol. II, p. 153.
18. Ehrlich and Morgenroth, *Collected Papers*, vol. II, p. 154.
19. Bordet, J., *Ann. Inst. Pasteur* 13:225, 1899; *Bordet Studies* pp. 142–164.
20. Kraus, R. *Wien. klin. Wochenschr.* 10:736, 1897.
21. Bordet, J., *Ann. Inst. Pasteur* 13:273, 1899; *Bordet Studies* pp. 165–185.
22. Bordet, note 21, p. 278.
23. Bordet, note 21, p. 281.
24. Bordet, note 21, p. 282.
25. Bordet, note 21, p. 288.

26. Landsteiner, K. and Reich, M., *Wien. klin. Rundschau* 19:568, 1905. See also Landsteiner, in *Handbuch der Biochemie,* C. Oppenheimer, ed., Vol. I., Jena, Gustav Fischer, 1910.

27. Ehrlich, P. and Morgenroth, J., *Berl. klin. Wochenschr.* 36:481, 1899; *Collected Papers* vol. II, pp. 165–172.

28. For a discussion of the broad implications of these terminological differences that represented in fact incommensurable languages, see Silverstein, A.M., *Cell. Immunol.* 97:173, 1986.

29. This is an adaptation of Emil Fischer's famous lock-and-key metaphor, coined to describe the interaction of enzyme with substrate. Ehrlich would apply it repeatedly to describe the antigen–antibody interaction.

30. Müller-Eberhard, H.J., *Advances Immunol.* 8:1. 1968; Mayer, M.M., *Proc. Nat. Acad. Sci. U.S.* 69:2954, 1972; Mayer, M.M., *Complement* 1:2, 1984.

31. Ehrlich, P., The Croonian Lecture, *Proc. Roy. Soc. London,* 66:424, 1900; *Collected Papers* vol. II, pp. 178–195.

32. Bordet, J., *Ann. Inst. Pasteur* 14:257, 1900; *Bordet Studies,* pp. 186–216.

33. It has been suggested to me that this is a very Gallic stance; even worse than "damning with faint praise" is "damning by complete disregard."

34. Danysz, J. *Ann. Inst. Pasteur* 16:331, 1902.

35. Portier, P. and Richet, C., *C.R. Soc. Biol.* 54:170, 1902.

36. Bordet, note 32, p. 282.

37. Bordet and Gengou, note 3.

38. Gengou, O., *Ann. Inst. Pasteur* 16:734, 1902.

39. Pfeiffer, note 10.

40. Fraenkel, C. and Sobernheim, G., *Hyg. Rundschau* 4:97, 145, 1894.

41. Metchnikoff, note 11.

42. Ehrlich, P. and Morgenroth, J., *Berlin klin. Wochenschr.* 37:453, 1900; *Collected Papers* vol. II, pp. 205–212.

43. Landsteiner, K., *Centralbl. Bakt.* 25:549, 1899.

44. Metchnikoff, E., *Ann. Inst. Pasteur,* 13:737, 1899.

45. Metalnikoff, S., *Ann. Inst. Pasteur* 14:577, 1900.

46. von Dungern, E., *Münch. med. Wschr.* 46:1228, 1899.

47. Besredka, A., *Ann. Inst. Pasteur* 14:390, 1900.

48. Metchnikoff, E., *Ann. Institut Pasteur* 14:1, 1900.

49. Ehrlich and Morgenroth, note 42, *Collected Papers,* vol. II, p. 206.

50. Landsteiner, K., *Zentralbl. Bakteriol.* 27:357, 1900.

51. Ehrlich and Morgenroth, note 42, *Collected Papers II* p. 208.

52. Jerne, N.K., *Ann. Immunol. (Paris)* 125C:373, 1974.

53. The details of this anticipation of Jerne's network theory are discussed in Silverstein, A.M., *A History of Immunology,* New York, Academic Press, 1989, pp. 252–274.

54. Ehrlich, P. and Morgenroth, J., *Berl. klin. Wochenschr.* 37:681, 1900; *Collected Papers* vol. II, pp. 224–233.

55. Buchner, H. *Münch. med. Wschr.* 47:277, 1900.

56. Ehrlich and Morgenroth, Note 54, *Collected papers* vol. II, p. 227.

57. Ehrlich and Morgenroth, note 54, *Collected Papers* vol. II, p. 233.

58. Ehrlich, P., *Collected Studies in Immunity* (C. Balduan, transl.), New York, Wiley; London, Chapman and Hall, xi + 586 pp, 1906. This volume also includes studiea by Ehrlich's collaborators.

59. Ehrlich, P. and Morgenroth, J., *Berl. klin. Wochenschr.* 38:251, 1901; *Collected Papers* vol. II, pp. 246–255.

60. Ehrlich and Morgenroth, note 59, *Collected Papers* vol. II, p. 252.

61. Ehrlich, P. and Sachs, H., *Berl. klin. Wochenschr.* 39:492, 1902.

62. Metalnikoff, note 45.

63. Von Pirquet, C., *Allergie,* Berlin, Springer, 1910; English transl., *Allergy,* Chicago, American Medical Association, 1911; see also Silverstein, A.M., *Nature Immunol.* 1:453, 2000.

64. Kraus, note 20.

65. Gengou, note 38.

66. Portier and Richet, note 35.

67. Arthus, M., *C.R. Soc. Biol.* 55:817, 1903.

68. Bordet and Gengou, note 3.

69. von Pirquet, C. and Schick, B., *Das Serumkrankheit,* Vienna, Deuticke, 1906; English transl. *Serum Sickness,* Baltimore, Williams & Wilkins, 1951.

70. Ehrlich, P. and Morgenroth, J. *Berl. klin. Wochenschr.* 38:569, 598, 1901; *Collected Papers* vol. II, pp. 278–297.

71. See Morgenroth's review of these studies, *Arch. Int. Pharmacodynam.* 7:265, 1900.

72. The entire question of receptor specificity, antigenic cross-reactions, and selective absorption to sharpen the specificity of an antiserum is reviewed by von Dungern, E., in the Festschrift celebrating Ehrlich's 60th birthday, *Paul Ehrlich: Eine Darstellung Seines Wissenschaftlichen Wirkens,* Jena, Fischer, 1914, pp. 163–164.

73. Already in 1900, von Dungern (*Münch. med. Wochenschr.* 47:675, 1900; *Collected Studies* pp. 36–46) had hinted that there is an inverse relationship between the amount of antibody and of complement needed to effect a given degree of hemolysis. This appeared to have been overlooked, until it was more closely investigated and more fully quantitated by Morgenroth and Sachs in 1902 (*Berl. klin. Wochenschr.* 39:631, 1902; *Collected Studies,* pp. 250–266).

74. Bordet, J., *Ann. Inst. Pasteur* 15:303, 1901; *Bordet Studies,* pp. 228–240.

75. Ehrlich, P. and Marshall. H.T., *Berl. klin. Wochenschr.* 39:585, 1902; *Stud. Rockefeller Inst. Med. Res.* 2: 1904; *Collected Papers* vol. II, pp. 342–346.

76. The initial suggestion by sociologists of science (e.g., Thomas Merton, *"The normative structure of science,"* in *The Sociology of Science,* Chicago, University of Chicago Press, 1973, p. 267) and philosophers of science (e.g., Karl Popper, *The Logic of Scientific Discovery,* New York, Basic Books, 1959) was that science works most efficiently by agreement. This has given way to the more radical concepts of Thomas Kuhn (*The Structure of Scientific Revolutions,* Chicago, University of Chicago Press, 1970) and of Imre Lakatos (in *Criticism and the Growth of Knowledge,* Lakatos, I. and Musgrove, A., eds., London, Cambridge University Press, 1970) that highlight instead the heuristic value for science of disputes and inconsistencies.

77. *Bordet Studies,* note 1, p. 507.

78. For a more detailed discussion of Bordet's style and epistemological position, see E. Crist and A.I. Tauber, "Debating humoral immunity and epistemology: The rivalry of the immunochemists Jules Bordet and Paul Ehrlich," *J. Hist. Biol.* 30:321, 1997. (I think that Bordet would have been shocked to have been called an immunochemist.)

79. Bordet's "single complement" referred, of course, to a single *function* common to all immune interactions, and not to the congeries of components that would later be demonstrated to constitute the complement cascade; see note 30.

80. Bordet, J., *Traité de L'Immunité dans les Maladies Infectieuses,* 2nd ed., Paris, Masson, 1939.

81. Bordet, note 80, p. iv.

8

NEW SCIENTIFIC
CHALLENGES

Corpora non agunt nisi fixata.

Paul Ehrlich

One of the most curious phenomena in science is the frequent suggestion that a given discipline has finally solved all of its problems; there is little else left to do but perhaps some cleanup of minor details, and the next generation might as well seek other fields to conquer. This declaration of the end of a science is most often made explicitly by its own elder statesmen, who seem to imply that *their* work has provided the finishing touches, beyond which no significant advances can be expected. Thus, to cite but a few notable examples,[1] Lord Kelvin declared in the 1890s that it was all over in physics (just before the Einsteinian revolution); in 1968, Gunter Stent, in a series of lectures at the University of California, Berkeley,[2] declared that molecular biology had already peaked (this not long before the burst of activity that led to the human genome project and to genetic engineering); and both Macfarlane Burnet[3] and Niels Jerne[4] concluded in the 1960s that the clonal selection theory had pretty much solved all of immunology's problems (just before the immunobiological revolution).[5]

It would appear that after 1901, Paul Ehrlich had the same feeling about his contributions to immunology, although he never declared it explicitly. He had, after all, advanced his side-chain theory of antibody formation that was, in most immunological laboratories, the ruling paradigm that guided the planning of experiments and the interpretation of results. And he had, in his work on toxin–antitoxin and hemolysin-erythrocyte interactions, fairly well characterized the mechanisms by which these antibodies function. Aside from continuing his attempts to convert the residual nonbelievers (e.g., Elie Metchnikoff, Jules Bordet, Max von Gruber, and Svante Arrhenius), it is likely that Ehrlich felt that there was little left to do in immunology, and one ought to move on to address other important challenges. He would leave to his assistants Julius Morgenroth and Hans Sachs the residual "cleanup" work required in immunology.

Indeed, there is good reason to believe that Ehrlich felt that there was little else left to do in immunology even before his landmark studies with Morgenroth on immune hemolysis. In November 1899, he could say in a letter to a Dr. Clemens, "I did not have a chance to deal with this matter [the diazo reaction in urinalysis] in a chemical way, since I slipped in the last 10 years into immunological "hocus-pocus."[6]

We will review briefly those new areas of activity that Ehrlich entered, providing only a taste of his involvement in each. It must not be thought, however, that each phase of Ehrlich's scientific career ended sharply after he had begun to focus on a new problem; he would maintain an interest and even publish in areas of earlier involvement long after he had moved on to a different discipline, especially when the earlier work had been challenged.

CANCER RESEARCH

In his lengthy review of Ehrlich's tumor studies,[7] Hugo Apolant points out that of all the scientific fields to which Ehrlich contributed, only cancer research did not originate directly from his ideas about receptors. This is not to say, of course, that he did not eventually introduce receptors into his concept of the growth, rejection, and inhibition of tumors, as we shall see. Rather, it happened that soon after Ehrlich had completed his landmark studies of immune hemolysis with Julius Morgenroth (see Chapter 7), a number of generous donors made significant sums available to him for the support of cancer research. These had been stimulated by the intercession of Ehrlich's chief sponsor, Ministerial Director Friedrich Althoff, and by the former Mayor of Frankfurt, Dr. Franz Adickes, both of whom had collaborated in the initial establishment of Ehrlich's Institute. This is not to suggest that Ehrlich would "sell" himself to an inferior science: cancer research was in the air, it presented fascinating and important challenges, and Ehrlich was presumably ready for a new scientific venture. One knew that if Ehrlich turned his attention to a problem, he would bring to it his imaginative best, and he did not disappoint. In the autumn of 1901, he set up a cancer division within his institute, and recruited for it such individuals as Prowazek and Weidenreich intially, and then Embden and Apolant. This was to be a serious venture.

Ehrlich's approach to the study of the biology of tumors concentrated on the development of a library of transplantable tumors and the establishment of the rules that govern their acceptance in normal recipients, their growth, and their formation of metastases.[8] He developed the notion of tumor "virulence," analogous to the virulence of pathogenic organisms. As with pathogens, this characteristic could be measured by such factors as the dose required to achieve successful transfer, the rapidity of growth and invasiveness of the transplant, and its proclivity to seed metastases elsewhere in the recipient. He showed also that the "virulence" of many tumors could be enhanced significantly on repeated passage from animal to animal, whereas the virulence of other tumors (most notably sarcomas) was attenuated by exposure to elevated temperatures. Of great interest was the demonstration that the injection of a given tumor into an animal might lead to an apparent "immunity," wherein a second transplant of the same tumor resulted in little or no growth. At the outset, this was viewed by the Ehrlich group as a manifestation of the same type of immunological response that was seen following immunization with erythrocytes, but the absence of demonstrable circulating antitumor antibodies caused them to abandon this theory.

What factors determine the "take" of a tumor transplant and the rate at which it would subsequently grow? For Ehrlich, the answer had to be in the availability of appropriate nutrition in the new environment. This must perforce depend on receptors for each of the nutrients involved, which Ehrlich termed *nutri-receptors*. It will be recalled that in his side-chain theory, Ehrlich had insisted that antibodies are only special instances of the broad range of cell surface receptors required by a cell to transact its normal functions, including both the ingestion of nutrients and the interaction with dyes, drugs, toxins, and so on.

Thus, everything appeared to be explicable in terms of the presence or absence of receptors on the donor tumor, or the presence or absence of the required nutrients in the recipient of the tumor. A tumor that failed to grow in a new host must have failed to find adequate nutrition; those that grew well must have found a fertile "soil" in which to flourish. Again, the failure of second tumor transplants to thrive was attributed to the depletion by the initial transplant of those nutrients essential to tumor growth. Perhaps the concept was best illustrated by the explanation advanced by Ehrlich[9] to explain the fact that when certain carcinomas are transplanted, they are rapidly taken over by a minor sarcomatous contaminant, while the transplantation of mixtures of carcinoma and sarcoma cells invariably gives rise to pure sarcomatous growth.[10] This was explained[11] by the presence on the sarcoma cells of more appropriate receptors for those nutrients present in the recipient host than were possessed by the carcinoma cells.

Ehrlich's theory of the importance of nutritional factors in the development and growth of tumors had one immediate and important effect; it reinforced the growing impression that cancer cells are nothing more than normal cells gone astray. This was due to his suggestion[12] that the essence of tumor formation lies in avidity differences between cancer cells and normal cells; they are otherwise similar, and require the same nutrients for their growth. The side-chain theory thus predicted that the advantage of the tumor cell depends on one of two factors: either (a) it has more nutrient receptors than the normal cell does, or (b) its receptors are more avid than those of the normal cell. In either case, the tumor cell will be better nourished and therefore flourish more exuberantly.

Ehrlich termed this concept of nutritional inhibition of growth "athrepsia" (Gr. *trephein*, to nourish). He admitted that the idea was not new,[13] and cited an analogous theory advanced many years earlier by Louis Pasteur[14] to explain the mechanism of adaptive immunity, a theory that did not long survive. At a time when only live, attenuated pathogens were known to induce acquired immunity, Pasteur had suggested that, by analogy with bacterial growth in culture, the exhaustion of trace nutrients would inhibit further growth of the pathogen, and thus the infected or immunized animal would be rendered immune to further challenge. This concept, in the field of immunology, did not survive the discovery of phagocytosis and of immune (antibody) responses to inert toxins and dead bacteria. But Ehrlich's specific nutri-receptors gave athrepsia a new life in the context of tumor biology; however, not all researchers in the field accepted the concept.

One of the more interesting observations made during these tumor studies involved the transplantation of a mouse tumor into the rat.[15] The tumor would grow rapidly until about the 6th day, whereupon growth would suddenly cease and the tumor would be completely destroyed. However, excision of the tumor in the rat prior to its failure and passage of it back to the mouse would see it continue to flourish. The same process, zigzagging the tumor between rat and mouse, could be repeated for many generations. Ehrlich explained this according to his theory of athrepsia; the rat, being deficient in some of the nutritive elements required by this tumor, could only support its growth for a short period, whereas the mouse, possessing these nutrients in abundance, could support its growth indefinitely.

Ehrlich would later extend his theory of athrepsia to the survival or death of bacterial invasions of the body, and to the distribution of lesions during infection.[16] He suggested that the failure of an organism to survive in a given host, or to mutiply and cause disease in a given tissue, depends on the availability of appropriate nutrients. Thus, most species will not support infection by *Treponema pallidum,* but the monkey can be infected, although only in the skin and not by parenteral inoculation, suggesting that only this susceptible site can nourish the pathogen of syphilis. Again, fowlpox can be transferred from hen to pigeon, but after several passages in the pigeon can no longer be propagated back to the hen. Ehrlich suggested that this change is due to the stepwise loss (atrophy) of hen-specific receptors on the pathogen, while pigeon-specific receptors multiply.

Another fascinating aspect of the transplantation story is how early researchers developed experimental approaches involving *parabiotic* animal preparations. These involved rabbits, in studies by Sauerbruch and Heyde,[17] rats by Morpurgo,[18] and mice by Schöne.[19] Almost invariably, one member of the parabiotic pair would suffer a wasting disease, while the other grew. At first this was ascribed to a blood-induced "toxic anemia," wherein the stronger of the two overpowered the weaker, but Ehrlich suggested that it was yet another example of the workings of athrepsia. Here, the stronger party was supposedly able to monopolize the nutrients shared by the two, at the expense of the weaker member. Later studies by Hasek, Simonsen, Trentin, and others would confirm the broad utility of parabiotic preparations[20] and demonstrate that the wasting disease was the result of a purely immunological *graft-vs-host* reaction.[21]

It is worth recalling here a logical inconsistency in Ehrlich's theory of athrepsia that was alluded to in a somewhat different context in Chapter 5. Presumably, the receptors for nutrients should function in a manner similar to the receptors for toxins, which had provided the basis for his side-chain theory. But if the interaction of toxins with their specific receptors leads to their overproduction and release into the circulation as protective antibodies, why then should not the nutrient receptors respond similarly? If this were to occur, then "anti-nutrient" antibodies should appear in the blood able to "neutralize" the nutrients before they can reach and nourish the cell; this obviously does not happen. It was never adequately explained why nutri-receptors alone should be exempt from the process of receptor activation, overproduction, and shedding into the blood, and again it is curious that this inconsistency was not recognized by Ehrlich's opponents and used as a strong argument against his theory.

As we look back on the flurry of activity in cancer research that occurred during the first decade of this century, we cannot escape the conclusion that here, for the first time, Ehrlich's keen scientific intuition failed him. Studies on the acceptance and rejection of transplantable tumors were in progress in many laboratories, most notably in those of the Imperial Cancer Research Fund in London. Especially at the latter institution, it was repeatedly observed that after rejection of a tumor, transplantation of a second graft of that same tumor would invariably fail. However, when controls were run using normal tissues from the same donor for the initial sensitization, failure of the (second) tumor graft was seen also; obviously, it was something innate in the tissues of the donor rather than something peculiar to the tumor that caused the incompatibility.

Ehrlich, having advanced a theory of athrepsia, explained these results in its terms (i.e., in terms of the availability or exhaustion of nutrients and/or nutrient receptors). In London, E.F. Bashford and his colleagues chose to view this phenomenon in purely immunological terms.[22] In an era when immunological concepts were in the forefront, when anaphylaxis had become one of the popular topics of the time, and after Richet and Héricourt had suggested as early as 1895 the possibility of serotherapy for the treatment of cancer,[23] it is surprising that it was the oncologist Bashford rather than the immunologist Ehrlich who would provide an immunological explanation of tumor rejection. Thus, the results with tumor grafts were quickly generalized to cover the immunologic response to and rejection of *all* foreign tissues.

The same Georg Schöne (now removed from Frankfurt to Greifswald), who would summarize Ehrlich's theory of athrepsia (see note 11), published a remarkable book on tissue transplantation in 1912.[24] In it, he cited almost 500 references to transplantation studies (demonstrating the broad contemporary interest in the field), and even coined the term *"transplantation immunity."* Schöne condensed the results of these studies into six general rules that he believed underlay all of the phenomenology of transplantation:

1. Transplantation into a foreign species (heteroplastic = xenogeneic) invariably fails.
2. Transplantation into unrelated members of the same species (homoplastic = allogeneic) usually fails.
3. Transplantation of autografts almost invariably succeeds.

4. Using allografts, there is a primary take and then a delayed rejection of first grafts.
5. Second allografts undergo accelerated rejection in hosts that have rejected a primary from the same donor, or that have been immunized with tissue from from the tumor donor.
6. The closer the "blood relationship" between donor and recipient, the more likely the graft is to succeed.

Here, already in 1912, are the "laws of transplantation" substantially as they are understood today.[25] However, probably because tissue transplantation was tied to immunology by experimental oncologists and the results published primarily in their literature, it did not enter into mainstream immunological thought at that time. Indeed, even the original studies in the 1940s and early 1950s by Medawar and associates did not attract much attention in immunological circles. Medawar was a zoologist, and published in anatomy and pathology journals; only after the mid-1950s did his work begin to influence immunologists, and only then did he and the members of his group start to think of themselves as immunologists.[26] Had Paul Ehrlich not been so wedded to his theory of athrepsia, and had he been willing to consider the phenomena of tumor acceptance and rejection from a purely immunological point of view, the history of transplantation immunology would doubtless have developed far differently.

CHEMOTHERAPY

Just as 1901 saw a major shift in Ehrlich's interests from immunology to experimental oncology, so 1905 saw yet another shift, this time to chemotherapy.[27] We attributed the former shift to Ehrlich's probable feeling that his immunological theory and experiments had substantially solved the major outstanding problems in that field, and perhaps we were correct in this assumption. But the problems of experimental tumor research in 1905 were far from solved, although Ehrlich had surely made important contributions in this field. Perhaps Martha Marquardt was closer to the mark, in the context of this latter change of scientific direction, when she quotes Ehrlich as saying generously, "One must not stay in a field of work until the crops are completely brought in, but leave still some part of the harvest for the others."[28]

In any event, the challenges posed by infectious diseases remained in the forefront of early 20th-century medicine. The limitations of preventive vaccination, and especially of serotherapy, had become all too evident; immunology seemed ineffective in preventing or curing such important diseases as tuberculosis, syphilis, the gram-positive infections, and especially the parasitic diseases that ravaged much of the world. As early as New Year's Day, 1905, Ehrlich wrote to Ministerialdirektor Althoff that,

> I have, generally speaking, the impression that it is necessary that I concentrate all of my energy, consistent with my innate ability, to *chemical therapy*. Now is the moment to

confront the major types of illness (protozoan diseases) from the direction of chemical approaches, which are not very open to immunization therapy.[29]

Thus, when Frau Franziska Speyer wished to endow a research institute in memory of her late husband, Frankfurt banker Georg Speyer, it would not be an institute of cancer research (from which disease her husband had died) but an institute of chemotherapy![30] The Speyer Institute was built adjacent to Ehrlich's Royal Institute for Experimental Therapy, and Ehrlich managed both. He would say at its dedication,

> The aims of the new Speyer Haus follow different, though parallel, lines [from those of the Institute for Experimental Therapy]. Here too, the problem is to cure an organism infected by particular parasites by killing the parasites within the living organism, only this time not with the aid of the protective substances produced by the organism in acquired immunity, but with the aid of substances formed in the chemist's retort. The task of the new institute is thus the specific chemotherapy of infectious diseases. Simple reflection will show that this is bound to be a far more difficult issue than that of serum therapy. ... we are not so easily going to find such magic substances as antibodies which attack only the harmful agent.[31]

How was this new approach to be accomplished? Here, the full strength of Ehrlich's grounding in organic chemistry would come to the fore.[32] He had already demonstrated the quality of his chemical thinking in his side-chain theory and earlier in his work on the relationship between the chemical structure and the biological activity of dyestuffs. Now, the same approach would be employed; just as dyes could be acidophilic, basophilic, neurotropic, and so on, so might other chemicals be parasitotropic. Ehrlich would henceforth screen large numbers of compounds to determine which had an effect on parasites, and then use his organic-chemical imagination to design derivatives to enhance their parasiticidal effect while minimizing their toxicity for the host. Thus was a truly scientific chemotherapy founded. Its aim was, as Ehrlich would put it, to develop a *therapia magna sterilisans,* in which the drug would completely destroy the pathogen while fully sparing the tissues of the host.

Malaria

As early as 1891, and based on his extensive knowledge of the differential staining of cells by dyes, Ehrlich took note of the report that the plasmodia that cause malaria are strongly stained by methylene blue. Knowing that this dye is nontoxic in humans, he proposed to try it as a therapeutic agent in two cases of malaria present in Guttmann's clinic. The concept underlying this approach was that the dye appeared to be "parasitotropic" (in Ehrlich's terminology) and not "organotropic" in the human, and thus might exert a specific effect on the para-site. In the event, this chemical was found to yield clearly positive therapeutic results,[33] and the authors suggested that it might be employed profitably in con-junction with quinine therapy. However, in the absence of further cases of malaria locally, and because Ehrlich's attention was being drawn inexorably toward immunological research, the observation was not followed up.

Trypanosomiasis

The study of trypanosomes early in the 20th century was opened up by the demonstration by Laveran and Mesnil[34] that the disease could be studied in infected mice. This led to two observations that would assume much greater significance in future work on the prevention and therapy of certain infectious diseases. The first involved what was called at the time "serum-fastness" or "serum-resistance." This was seen in animals that had been partially cured of an infection, but then suffered a recurrence. The surviving trypanosomes were found to differ from the original strain, in that they could now infect an animal immune to the original strain. This was first interpreted by Ehrlich[35] as the disappearance from the original strain of organisms of a putative nutri-receptor "A" and its replacement by another nutrireceptor "B." Since it appeared that anti-trypanosomal antibodies are not directly cytotoxic, Ehrlich assumed that the antibody acted as an anti-nutri-receptor, thus interfering with the pathogen's nutrition. Thus, anti-"A" antibodies would inhibit "A"-type trypanosmes, but have no effect on "B"-type organisms. He gave the name *athrepsins* to these antibodies, and suggested that a trypanosome with multiple nutri-receptor types could only be damaged by antibodies capable of occupying (i.e., inhibiting the function of) all of these sites. It will be obvious that this phenomenon of "serum-fastness" has come to be recognized as antigenic variation, one of the many ways in which pathogens have learned to circumvent the inhibitions of the immune response, and one that has assumed great significance in modern efforts to develop efficacious vaccines against influenza and a number of tropical diseases.

The second observation stemming from trypanosomal research was the development of drug-resistant strains of the organism.[36] With repeated exposure to small doses of a drug such as atoxyl, a given strain of trypanosomes will soon become completely impervious to its action. Ehrlich called the receptors for these drugs "chemoreceptors." He suggested that in "drug-fast" strains the receptor does not disappear, but rather loses its avidity for the drug. Again, this phenomenon of the development of drug resistance has become an important issue in modern medicine, when antibiotics are so ubiquitous and overutilized.

Ehrlich continued his search for trypanocidal dyes, in collaboration with the visiting Japanese researcher Kiyoshi Shiga.[37] They developed the agent called trypan red, much more effective in curing trypanosomal infection, but still somewhat too toxic to be employed in the human. However, this observation was accompanied by a finding that would assume great future significance in pharmacology; the compound was not trypanocidal *in vitro,* but only in the infected host. This meant that the active substance was some metabolic intermediate formed by the action of the host on the original compound. Work on other derivatives of these benzidine dyes was extended by Mesnil and Nicolle, who developed the even more effective trypanocide trypan blue.[38]

The French investigators had shown that inorganic arsenious acid was trypanocidal, but it also was quite toxic to the host. Ehrlich would now investigate organic arsenic compounds. He had quite early tried the arsenic-containing substance atoxyl (*p*-aminophenylarsonic acid) on trypanosomes, but found it ineffective on the strains of organisms that he had available, and so he let it drop. But when atoxyl was shown to be effective against other strains of trypanosomes, he returned to it with good results. However, atoxyl proved too toxic for practical use, and Ehrlich showed that derivatives of this compond, such as acetylarsanilic acid (Ehrlich's preparation 306, given the tradename arsacetin) and arsenophenylglycine (preparation 418) might be equally or even more effective, while at the same time being less toxic for the host.

Spirochetal Diseases—Syphilis

Until 1903, syphilis was thought to be restricted only to humans; then Roux and Metchnikoff described the infection of chimpanzees,[39] and in 1905 Schaudinn identified the causative agent, *Treponema pallidum*.[40] Since Schaudinn was known to suspect a relationship between trypanosomes and spirochetes, Ehrlich felt that it might be useful to extend his experiments with arsenicals to syphils.[41] In Berlin, Paul Uhlenhuth had already been experimenting with atoxyl for the treatment of chicken spirillosis, another disease caused by spirochetes; Uhlenhuth would later dispute with Ehrlich the priority for initiating the chemotherapy of syphilis.

Over the course of the next four to five years, some 300 additional compounds were tested for efficacy and safety. Some were chemicals submitted from the laboratories at the Hoechst Chemical Company, with whom Ehrlich had a contractual arrangement for the commercial exploitation of any agents deemed worthwhile. Many compounds were synthesized at the suggestion of Ehrlich himself, who would choose a promising starting material and then suggest the preparation of derivatives; he might even suggest to chemists Alfred Bertheim and Ludwig Benda which substitution or condensation reaction they should employ to attain the desired product!

In March 1909, a new Japanese colleague, Sahashiro Hata, arrived in Frankfurt, sent to Ehrlich by his old friend from Koch's institute in Berlin, Kitasato. Hata worked tirelessly, testing one compound after another to determine its action both on trypanosomal infections as well as on the spirochetal infections syphilis, chicken spirillosis, and relapsing fever. Then, in early June 1909, Hata tested a new compound, number 606, and found that a single dose of only 3.5 mg/kg would completely cure birds suffering from chicken spirillosis. The more severe test of the drug, on relapsing fever, proved equally promising. Hata would conclude that, "Dihydroxy-diamino-arsenobenzene [preparation 606, soon to be given the tradename Salvarsanl consistently displays protective and curative activity in relapsing fever in mice and rats; the successes which I have recorded with this compound surpass all those achieved previously." Morover, as respects toxicity, Hata noted that "unpleasant side effects involving the nervous system (such as tremor, chorea, and amaurosis in particular), which are easily caused by other chemical agents, were not once observed in animals treated with [606]."[42] Hoechst immediately filed a patent on 606, but in it mentioned only its beneficial effects on the spirochete of relapsing fever.

But the application of this new drug to syphilis was not long in coming. It was quickly shown to cure an active case of syphilitic inflammation of the rabbit cornea, and then the syphilitic ulcers that accompany scrotal infection in the rabbit.[43] Cautiously, Ehrlich had the compound tested and retested, and finally, in September 1909, Ehrlich proposed a clinical trial in "hopeless cases of late syphilis" in patients at a lunatic asylum run by his colleague Konrad Alt. The results were highly promising, and it was soon found that the drug was even more effective in cases of recently acquired syphilis. One trial after another showed the new drug to be effective in the treatment of syphilis, and soon the demand for it exceeded the production capacity of Hoechst.

Full recognition of this great advance in therapeutics occurred not only in the press worldwide, but formally at the 82nd Congress of German Natural Scientists and Physicians at Königsberg, where Ehrlich was received "to unbroked applause." The Dean of German dermatologists and venereologists, Privy Councilor Professor Albert Neisser, reviewing the history of the struggle against syphilis, could say,

> it is because we now know that Ehrlich's new compound is precisely such a wonderful weapon against syphilis that our sense of gratitude and admiration for the man is so great and heartfelt. ... If syphilis is justifiably referred to as the scourge of mankind, then Ehrlich may with equal justification be called the benefactor of mankind.[44]

THE LAST YEARS

Just as Ehrlich had been forced to defend his immunological offerings, so was he challenged on his chemotherapy, especially on Salvarsan. He had issued very precise instructions on the use of Salvarsan, cautioning about dosage, about the sterility and purity of the water employed for its solution, about the care to to be exercised to ensure that nothing be injected outside the vein, and that the treatment not be employed in cases of neurosyphilis or in patients with certain organ failures or with diabetes. Nevertheless, report after report was made of failure of cure, of activation of neural symptoms, of infection, and even of death, and in each instance Ehrlich had to track down the problem and expose the true cause.[45]

The challenge to his Salvarsan therapy came especially forcefully from a Berlin dermatologist Richard Dreuw. This individual actually achieved a degree of fame in leading the attack on the famous Ehrlich, and mobilized a variety of forces behind it, including some from right-wing political factions who were openly anti-Semitic. Dreuw even instigated a debate on Salvarsan in the German Reichstag. In the end, Ehrlich made the point in 1914 that, in view of the staggering death rate from syphilis and of the fact that well over 1,000,000 people had been treated with Salvarsan, even if there had actually been 275 deaths due to the drug (a fact that Ehrlich disputed), the benefits of treatment must far outweigh its harm. As with his immunological disputes, Ehrlich maintained in his file *Polemics* a thick folder labeled "Anti-Dreuw."[46]

In spite of all attacks, Salvarsan and its successor Neosalvarsan received world-wide acceptance and acclaim, as indicated above. It will be recalled that Ehrlich, having been nominated for a Nobel Prize for his immunology each year starting in 1901, finally received this coveted award in 1908 (see Chapter 5 for the story of Svante Arrhenius's intervention with the Nobel Committee). Then, starting in 1913, he was once again nominated, this time for his contributions to chemotherapy in general, and to Salvarsan therapy of syphilis in particular. In his review of the Nobel Prizes in physiology, Liljestrand has concluded that Ehrlich would probably have received a second Prize, had he lived long enough.[47]

Paul Ehrlich died on August 20, 1915. He was buried in the Jewish Cemetery of Frankfurt, with a Star of David on one side of his gravesite, and the staff of Aesculapius on the other. His published obituary read in part,

> In you, Paul Ehrlich, we have lost one of the worthies of the heroic age of experimental therapeutic research; you were a king in the realm of a science which you yourself founded, and a teacher to innumerable researchers around the world who were proud to have studied under you. For you made disciples in an almost unprecedented way, and you became the *magister mundi* in medical science. Now you can rest from your difficult but successful labors, having completed an important mission in the furtherance of man's knowledge and resources. *Ave, pia anima.*[48]

Ehrlich's institute and the Speyer Haus were located in Frankfurt am Main on Sandhofstrasse. In 1912, this street was renamed Paul Ehrlich Strasse in his honor. Then, in 1938, in the midst of their virulent anti-Semitic campaign, the Nazis erased the name of Ehrlich from the street and from all other records; the name was "rehabilitated" in Germany after the end of World War II. But the name had lived on elsewhere in the Western world. When Hedwig Ehrlich fled Nazi Germany and found refuge in the United States in 1941, the American Medical Association held a reception at the Waldorf-Astoria hotel in New York to honor Ehrlich and his widow. The Surgeon General of the United States, Dr. Thomas Parran, gave the ceremonial address, ranking Ehrlich alongside the greatest doctors of the age. Some years later, at a celebration of the centenary of Ehrlich's birth in 1954, Sir Alexander Fleming said that

> Ehrlich's discovery of Salvarsan for the treatment of syphilis in 1909 marked the beginning of scientific chemotherapy. ... Paul Ehrlich is dead. It was not granted to him to witness the victory parade of antibacterial chemotherapy, the science which he founded. ... We are all humble and loyal disciples of the great man, and I honor his memory.[49]

NOTES AND REFERENCES

1. A more extensive discussion of this phenomenon can be found in Silverstein, A.M., *Hist. Sci.* 37:407, 1999.
2. Stent, G.S., *The Coming of the Golgen Age: A View of the End of Progress,* Garden City, NY, Natural History Press, 1969; see also Stent's *The Paradoxes of Progress,* San Francisco, W.H. Freeman, 1978.

3. This declaration was made by Burnet at the international symposium on *Molecular and Cellular Aspects of Antibody Formation* organized by Jaroslav Šterzl in Prague, Czechoslovakia, in 1964, attended by this author.

4. Jerne, N.K., "Summary: Waiting for the end," in *Antibodies: Cold Spring Harbor Symp. Quant. Biol.,* 32:591–603, 1967; see also Jerne's "The complete solution of immunology," *Austral. Ann. Med.,* 4:347, 1969.

5. For details on what I have termed elsewhere "the immunobiological revolution," see Silverstein, A.M., *Cell. Immunol.* 132:515, 1991.

6. Rockefeller Archives Center, *Ehrlich Papers,* 650 Eh 89, (henceforth *RAC Ehrlich Papers*) Box 6, Copirbuch IV, pp. 59–60; Beate Hirsch translation in *RAC Ehrlich Papers,* Box 55, folder 3. The term used by Ehrlich was *Immunitätszauber,* translated by Hirsch as "immunological hocus-pocus," but also possibly intended to convey "the lure of immunology."

7. Apolant, H., in the Festschrift for Ehrlich's 60th birthday, *Paul Ehrlich: Eine Darstellung Seines Wissenschaftlichen Wirkens,* Jena, Fischer, 1914, pp. 361–378 (henceforth *Ehrlich Festschroft*).

8. A full discussion of this study of the phenomenology of tumor transplants will be found in Apolant, *Ehrlich Festschrift,* note 7. One of the surviving benefits of these studies was the development of the Ehrlich ascites tumor, still employed today in tumor experiments.

9. Ehrlich, P. and Apolant, H., *Zentralbl. allg. Pathol. pathol. Anat.* 17:513, 1906.

10. Apolant, H., *Z. Krebsforsch.* 4:251, 1908.

11. A complete discussion of this and other presumed manifestations of nutritional factors will be found in Schöne, G., *Ehrlich Festschrift,* (note 7), pp. 379–408.

12. Ehrlich, P., *Arb. Inst. Exper. Ther. Frankfurt* 1:77–102, 1906; *Z. ärzt. Fortbldg.* 3:205–213, 1906; *Collected Papers* vol. II, pp. 493–511.

13. Ehrlich, P., *Z. Krebsforsch.* 5:59, 1907; *Collected Papers* vol. II, pp. 512–526.

14. Pasteur, L., Chamberland, C., and Roux, E., *C.R. Acad. Sci.* 90:239, 1880.

15. Ehrlich, note 13.

16. Ehrlich, P., *Beiträge zur experimentellen Pathologie und Chemotherapie,* Leipzig, Akad. Verlagsges., 1909.

17. Sauerbruch, F. and Heyde, M., *Z. exper. Pathol. Ther.* 6:33, 1909.

18. Morpurgo, B., *Münch. med. Wochenschr.* 55:2447, 1908. Morpurgo would ring some interesting changes in his studies of parabiosis; see, e.g., Morpurgo, *Ergebn. wiss. Med. Leipzig* 2:53, 1910–11.

19. Schöne, G., *Die Heteroplastische und Homöoplastische Transplantation,* Berlin, Springer, 1912.

20. See e.g., the papers by Simonsen, M. and Jensen, E. (p. 214–236) and by Trentin, J. (pp. 207–213), in *Biological Problems of Grafting,* Albert, F. and Medawar, P.B., eds., Oxford, Blackwell, 1959; also Hašek, M., Lengerová, A., and Hraba, T., *Advances Immunol.* 1:1, 1962.

21. Billingham, R.E., Brent, L., and Medawar, P.B., *Ann. N.Y. Acad. Sci.* 59:409, 1955; Trentin, J.J., *Proc. Soc. Exp. Biol. Med.* 92:688, 1956; Simonsen, M., *Acta Path. Microbiol. Scand.* 40:480, 1957. See also, Brent, L., *History of Transplantation,* San Diego, Academic Press, 1997.

22. See the *Annual Reports of the Imperial Cancer Research Fund,* 1903–1910; a history of the early years and contributions of this institution will be found in Austoker, J., *The History of the Imperial Cancer Research Fund 1902–1986,* London, Oxford University Press, 1988.

23. Richet, C. and Héricourt, J., *C.R. Acad. Sci.* 120:948, 1895.

24. Schöne, note 19.

25. The knowledge of the mechanisms of tissue transplantation were further advanced by E.E. Tyzzer in a broad review "Tumor Immunity" (*J. Cancer Res.* 1:125, 1916) by J.B. Murphy (*Monogr. Rockefeller Inst. Med. Res.* No. 21, 1926), and finally and most notably by Peter B. Medawar and his colleagues R.E. Billingham and L. Brent (see Medawar, *Harvey Lect.* 52:144, 1957 and Brent, *A History of Transplantation,* note 21).

26. The importance of these early transplantation biologists is discussed in further detail in Brent, *A History of Transplantation* note 21, and in Silverstein, A.M., *A History of Immunology,* New York, Academic Press, 1989, pp. 275–295.

27. This is not to imply that Ehrlich ceased all interest in immunology after 1901, or that he had done no work in cancer research after 1905. These were, each in its own time, his chief preoccupation.

28. M. Marquardt, *Paul Ehrlich,* London, Heinemann, 1949, pp. 115–116.

29. Ehrlich letter to Althoff, 1/1/1905, Rockefeller Archives Center, *RAC Ehrlich Papers,* box 10, file: "Briefe von Hedwig u. Paul Ehrlich an Friedrich Althoff," pp. 82–83.

30. It is possible that the decision toward chemotherapy was instigated solely by Frau Speyer's brother-in-law the chemist Professor Ludwig Darmstaedter, who organized the bequest. However, it is doubtful that this direction would have been taken had Ehrlich still been fully committed to cancer research rather than in active transition to the search for new drugs.

31. Ehrlich's address at the dedication of the Speyer Haus, *Collected Papers* vol. III, pp. 42–52.

32. In his Introductory Overview of Ehrlich's contributions to chemistry and biochemistry in the *Ehrlich Festschrift* (note 7), Professor R. Willstätter passes in revue the full extent of Ehrlich's chemical genius, pp. 411–416.

33. Guttmann, P. and Ehrlich, P., *Berl. klin. Wochenschr.* 28:953, 1891; *Collected Papers* vol. III, pp. 15–20.

34. Laveran, A. and Mesnil, F., *Ann. Inst. Pasteur* 15:673, 1901.

35. Ehrlich, P., *Berlin klin. Wschr.* 44:233, 280, 310, 341, 549, 1907; *Collected Papers* vol. III, pp. 81–105.

36. Ehrlich, P., *Verh. Berlin Med. Ges.* 38(part 2):35, 1908; *Collected Papers* vol. III, pp. 81–105.

37. Ehrlich P. and Shiga, K., *Berl. klin. Wschr.* 41:329, 362, 1904; *Collected Papers* vol. III, pp. 24–37.

38. Mesnil, F. and Nicolle, M. *Ann. Inst. Pasteur* 20:513, 1906.

39. Roux, E. and Metchnikoff, E., *Ann. Inst. Pasteur* 17:809, 1903.

40. Schaudinn, F. and Hoffmann, E., *Arb. Reichsgesundheitsamte* 22:527, 1905.

41. Cited by Bäumler, E., *Paul Ehrlich: Scientist for Life,* New York, Holmes & Meier, 1984, p. 126.

42. Quoted by Bäumler, *Paul Ehrlich,* note 41, p. 148.

43. These and other results are discussed in Ehrlich, P. and Hata, K., *Die Chemotherapie der Spirillosen,* Berlin, Springer, 1910; *Collected papers* vol. III, pp. 114–161 and 251–281.

44. Neisser, A. Speech at the 82nd Kongress der Deutsche Naturforscher und Ärzte, Königsberg, September 20, 1910, quoted by Bäumler, *Paul Ehrlich,* note 41, pp. 166–167.

45. The disputes over Salvarsan are discussed in some detail in Marquardt, *Paul Ehrlich,* note 28, pp. 188–206, and in Bäumler, *Paul Ehrlich,* note 41, pp. 175–210.

46. *RAC Ehrlich Papers,* Box 3, folder 17.

47. Liljestrand, G., "The Prize in Physiology," in *Nobel, the Man and his Prizes,* Stockholm, The Nobel Foundation, 1950, pp. 135–316. See also Jokl, E., "Paul Ehrlich—Man and Scientist" in the centennial celebration of Ehrlich's birth, *Bull. N. Y. Acad. Med.* 30:968, 1954.

48. Quoted by Bäumler, *Paul Ehrlich,* note 41, p. 148.

49. Quoted by Bäumler, *Paul Ehrlich,* note 41, pp. 234–235.

9

EHRLICH'S SCIENTIFIC STYLE

Bei Ehrlich lernte man arbeiten.
Georg Schöne[1]

Much has been written about the qualities that contribute to the making of a great scientist. In considering those who have distinguished themselves by a single significant discovery or concept, little can be said specifically, save perhaps for Louis Pasteur's famous dictum that "success favors the prepared mind." But for those whose entire scientific lifetime has been characterized by success after success—a Pasteur, a Koch, a Metchnikoff, or an Ehrlich—that and much more can be said. Now we may explore the question of temperament, of character, of training, of leadership, and even of obsession: in short, those qualities that contribute to what may be termed *scientific style.*

The principal aim of this chapter will be to explore some of the factors that contributed to Paul Ehrlich's scientific style, and to attempt to measure the extent to which these affected his approach to his science and his fellow scientists. At a somewhat deeper level, these are the factors that guide the individual in his choice of subject, in his interpretation of his data, in the type of speculations that he will permit himself, and even in the manner in which he runs his laboratory. It will be recognized that one or another aspect of this question has been touched on in each of the preceding chapters, as Ehrlich's many contributions have been passed in review. The reader is referred to the introduction to Chapter 5, where some of the more general features of scientific style were mentioned, including some of the epistemological and psychological differences that may distinguish one style from another.

A SCIENTIST'S OBSESSION

Perhaps more than any other scientist of his day, Ehrlich applied a single precept to every field into which he ventured and reaped in each a bountiful harvest. This was the idea, arrived at while still a medical student, that every physiological process depends on the initial interaction of some substance with a preformed receptor. Moreover, he would insist that this interaction is characterized by specificity, furnished by the stereochemical "fit" of the two components, as a key activates its proper lock. We saw earlier that Ehrlich developed this idea in the context of histological staining, wherein certain dyes interact only with certain cell types, presumably determined by the chemistry involved. Indeed, the notion is implicit in the names he gave to the several types of blood leukocytes that he described, the *eosinophile* (eosin [acid] lover), *basophile,* and *neutrophile.*

Thenceforth, Ehrlich would apply this concept to all manner of biological phenomena, each time following its lead into promising experiments with interesting and often valuable results. In immunology, his receptor theory led to the solution of the problem of assaying toxins and antitoxins; to the understanding that antibody formation is a natural *and inherent* physiological process; to the explanation of immunological specificity; to the first suggestion of independent *domains* on antibodies and antigens; and to the conclusion that the antigen-receptor interaction might trigger the activation of the cell bearing that receptor on its surface. Here was a concept that would appear and reappear in many different contexts throughout the development of the discipline of immunology.

His receptor theory appeared also in Ehrlich's work in experimental oncology. In this instance, however, it assumed a somewhat different form. Now it had to do directly with cell nitrition, in his theory of *athrepsia.* All cells were assumed to have *nutri-receptors,* which permit them to enjoy the benefit of the various nutrients on which their well-being depends. Ehrlich viewed the resistance or susceptibility of the host to tumor transplants as depending on the balance between the availability of certain required nutrients in the host and the presence of the appropriate receptors on the tumor cells. Although this concept did not pan out in the long run, it did prove to be heuristically valuable in Ehrlich's hands, in that it stimulated a variety of interesting experiments whose results would further progress in the field. This same theory of athrepsia would appear again in another guise, in Ehrlich's work on parasitic infections. He would explain the development of resistant strains of pathogens in terms of the acquisition of different nutri-receptors, a notion that resonates well with the modern understanding of the adaptive devices of pathogens as expressed in antigenic drift, antigenic shift, and drug resistance.

Finally, it was in his application of the concept of receptors to chemotherapy that Ehrlich realized perhaps his greatest and longest-lasting success. He sought to develop those toxic chemical compounds that could attach to receptors on the surface of the pathogen to effect its destruction, while unable to attach to the cells of the host due to the absence of such receptors. Here would be the specific chemotherapeutic agent, the perfect magic bullet that would achieve Ehrlich's ultimate aim, a *therapia magna sterilisans.*

It is clear that this preoccupation—indeed, obsession[2]—with receptors provided a continuity of approach that in Ehrlich's hands made him a leader in many fields. It contributed to his being named a "father" of the field of hematology,[3] his recognition as one of the founders of the discipline of immunology,[4] as a significant contributor to experimental oncology,[5] and as the founder of scientific pharmacology.[6] But even Ehrlich would have admitted that a guiding precept alone is not sufficient to ensure success. He would add to this what he called "The Four Big G's": *Geduld, Geschick, Geld,* and *Glück* (patience, ability, money, and luck).

A CHEMIST'S APPROACH

From his earliest days as a medical student, Ehrlich was attracted by the variety of highly colored dyes that poured forth from the growing German dye industry. He would, in later life, establish close ties to synthetic organic chemists in the industry, would hire several at his Frankfurt Institute, and would discuss molecular structure and function in many of his letters. He would not only propose the synthesis of special dye derivatives, but would even make suggestions about which reactions to employ to achieve the desired result. As he would say later,[7] he could "see" in his mind's eye the three-dimensional structure of a complicated compound. This disposition to think in organic chemical terms would exert a strong influence on both his immmunology and his chemotherapy.

We saw in Chapters 5 to 7 that Ehrlich's background in organic chemistry almost enforced the several conclusions he reached about antigens and antibodies. First, as a thinker in chemical terms, Ehrlich could not possibly accept Jules Bordet's proposal that antigens might interact with antibodies in a purely physical, adsorptive manner. He would insist that only a chemical interaction could provide both the force and the specificity to satisfy the interaction phenomena that the immune system manifested; a physical interaction could not, in his view, possibly fulfill the requirements of the data, and provide the specificity inherent in the interaction of a lock with its key.

Next, Ehrlich held that each biological molecule must be composed of *side-chains* like a complex organic molecule, each responsible for one or another function. These might serve for attachment to a receptor (the *haptophore,* the active site on the receptor itself) or as the effector of some physiological function (the *toxophore* group on a toxin or the *zymophore* group on a complement). He would picture these groups as he did the various attachments that could be added to a benzene molecule: a carboxyl or sulfonic acid group to increase aqueous solubility; an aliphatic group to increase solubility in organic solvents; an amino group to permit diazotization and coupling; or a hydroxyl group to permit esterification.

Finally, Ehrlich's exposure to organic chemistry enforced the view that all molecular interactions are tight and irreversible, like the condensation reactions of organic chemistry. He could not agree with Arrhenius's view that the interaction of toxin with antitoxin might be reversible, and indeed none of the *in vitro* interaction then available (hemolysin fixation to erythrocytes, the fixation of complement, the precipitin reaction, or bacterial agglutination by specific antibody) appeared to manifest the slightest degree of reversibility.

We must not imagine, however, that his proclivities toward chemical thinking diminished in any respect Ehrlich's approach to clinical medicine. As we go through his work on dyes, on tuberculin, on ricin and abrin, on diphtheria toxin–antitoxin interaction, and on pharmacology, it is amazing how he always returned to the clinical value of the work. Thus, he saw in fluorescein an approach to ocular physiology; in abrin a treatment for trachoma; in tuberculin a potential therapy; and in chemicals an approach to the cure of some of the most important diseases that afflict humanity. His introduction of quantitative methods into immunology was, in part, an attempt to understand the biology involved, but in the main an effort to improve the treatment of diphtheria and tetanus, among others.

THE RESPONSE TO CRITICISM

It is very difficult to understand why some scientists seem to maintain an allegiance to the validity of an idea long after its support has become, by general consent, unreasonable. We saw this phenomenon among a generation of immunochemists after the apparent victory of the immunobiological clonal selection theory; Felix Haurowitz went to his grave awaiting the vindication of instructionist theories of antibody formation,[8] and Alain Bussard still to this day awaits proof of the inadequacy of clonal selection.[9] But if adherence to a discipline's ruling paradigm is strong, even stronger will be one's adherence to *one's own* theory and one's own data that support it. Sometimes the explanation lies in nationalistic roots, as in the dispute about the basic nature of immunity, between the (predominantly French) cellularists and the (predominantly German) humoralists.[10] In regard to the excessive defense of one's own data, the most likely explanation rests, in all probability, so deep in the psyche of the individual as to defy ready analysis. But if the causes of this phenomenon are inaccessible for the most part, its consequences are often readily apparent.

Paul Ehrlich was one who, once he had gathered data on a problem and interpreted it in a certain way, seemed overly sensitive to any challenge to the validity either of the data themselves or his interpretation of them. This stance was not so evident in his early days. This was probably due in part to his youth and modest position in the world of science, but must in great measure be because he was breaking new ground with his histologic staining studies and his hematology, fields in which there were few to challenge him. But, even then, his self-assurance and willingness to innovate and to challenge foreshadowed a self-confidence and even an egotism regarding his science and its worth.

When Ehrlich ventured into immunology, however, he encountered many other investigators with views and personalities as strong as his own. As is so often the case, the conflicts stemmed less from questions of the validity of the data than from the manner in which these data were interpreted. Thus, Ehrlich would contest with Metchnikoff the relative importance of circulating antibodies and phagocytic cells in affording protection against infection; with Jules Bordet over the basis of immunological specificity and complement function; with Max Gruber over the validity of his side-chain theory and the nature of the neutralization of toxin by antitoxin; and with Svante Arrhenius over the question of whether the toxin–antitoxin interaction is or is not reversible. Ehrlich would later defend with passion his chemotherapeutic studies against attack, especially against the suggestion that his salvarsan was either dangerous to use or else ineffective.

It will not be necessary to repeat here the details of the various conflicts in which Ehrlich engaged with one or another opponent. Suffice it to say that he pursued each of them with vigor, never seeming to understand how *anyone* could have found fault with his analyses, theories, or predictions. However, one can detect differences in the way that he presented his position and attacked that of the antagonist, depending on the level of his esteem. Thus, he was always extremely polite in criticising Bordet,[11] somewhat less so in his words about Arrhenius,[12] and caustic in his treatment of Gruber, whom he appeared to have cordially detested. Thus, he could say about Gruber that "he knows [the field] merely from literary studies. Against such critics, I am in the unpleasant position of a man who is compelled to discuss colors with the blind."[13] He would say later, in desperation about Gruber's attacks, that "my position is like that of a chess player who, even though his game is won, is forced by the obstinacy of his opponent to carry on move by move until the final 'mate.'"[14]

In his own institute, however, Ehrlich was often less inhibited. He kept a large file labeled "POLEMICS,"[15] with notes and outlines covering each of his ongoing disputes. In addition, he would continually harp, in his notes to institute colleagues and his letters to friends, on the one that currently engaged him the most. Thus, a very small sample of his *Blöke*[16] to assistants within the institute included:

> To Morgenroth, 1900: "I have thought about the matter and would consider it very unwise, if we were to leave the lysin field now and let someone else harvest the cream. That would be a free meal for Bordet now."[17]
>
> To Morgenroth, June 1901: "The main thing is to finish the anti-Bordet work."[18]
>
> To self, June 1901: "New evidence against Bordet."[19]
>
> To Marx, Morgenroth, and Sachs, April 1902: "We have to do an anti-Gruber experiment in which only a minimal amount of serum is used."[20]
>
> To Morgenroth–Sachs, April 1902: "Perhaps Korschun could work on. ... More important is that he continue with all energy the anti-Metchnikoff matter."[21]
>
> To Marx, 1902: "I wanted to discuss with you. ... I think that the Pasteur people are preparing a similar attack and I'd like to beat them to the punch."[22]
>
> To Morgenroth, August 1902: "I was just thinking how much has to be done in the next two short weeks: 1) anti-Metchnikoff; 2) anti-Besredka."[23]
>
> To Sachs, no date: "It is high time for the publication of the Anti-Danysz. It will lose its significance if we sit on it too long."[24]

In a similar manner, whatever preoccupied him at the moment would be mentioned again and again in his letters to friends and sometimes even to seemingly casual correspondents. Thus, during the course of his defense against the various opponents of his concepts, we come across the following fairly representative examples:

> To Salomonsen, February 1899: "[we have] the phagocytic theory by the jugular."[25]
>
> To Gabritschewsky, February 1899: "The Pasteurians are *very* angry with me."[26]
>
> To Weigert, 1899: Ehrlich asks for comments on the draft of the second hemolysin paper. He "had to write it, since Bordet took over his [Ehrlich's] last results without credit. He naturally cut me out absolutely."[27]
>
> To Williamm Welch, 1899: "Your comments on Bordet. ... It's all Metchnikoff, of course."[28]
>
> To August Wassermann, early 1900: "Our common friend [Behring] is up in arms ... his obsession to topple the toxoid and side-chain theory."[29]
>
> To William Bulloch, November 1902: "Recently, Metchnikoff has not had many scientific triumphs."[30]
>
> To Theobald Smith, May 1904: In discussing a paper by Arrhenius and Madsen, "This is a true cuckoo's egg the authors have put into the immunity nest."[31]
>
> To Christian Herter, October 1904: "The dispute with Arrhenius continues, but I am not letting up. We blow out each of his eggs that he puts into our immunological nest."[32]
>
> To Ludwig Darmstädter, February 1910: "Madsen is an amiable, dear *Mensch,* and I can only regret that that fathead Arrhenius has so long opposed us."[33]

It will be apparent that Ehrlich took all challenges to his ideas very much to heart; in some cases, he almost appeared to take the challenge personally, as though he had been accused of practicing "bad science," or what might have seemed equally derogatory, foolishness. Given such "insults," and his supreme self-confidence, it is no wonder that he not only harped continuously on these challenges, but planned experiments specifically to counter them. One also must wonder whether Ehrlich's experience of having lost his share of the antitoxin profits to Behring (see Chapter 6) did not instill in him a more proprietary feeling about his scientific accomplishments. He would for years revisit again and again in his letters this feeling of betrayal by Behring. Finally, in a letter to Minsterialdirektor Althoff as late as 1906, he would say, "In the diphtheria campaign ... a constant scientific struggle between Behring and me resulted, from which I finally emerged victor, to be sure, but as a Pyrrhic victor, entirely exhausted, exaspirated, and warn out."[34]

The manner in which Ehrlich responded so strongly to criticism by answering not only with polemic, but also with experiment, has attracted the attention of many of Ehrlich's admirers and a number of observers of the sociology of science as well. Georg Gaffky commented on the importance of Ehrlich's opponents,

> It must appear very lucky in looking back on progress in immunology that the side-chain theory was not immediately fully accepted without opposition. The ensuing objections and debates caused Ehrlich and his students to perform a long series of magnificent experiments, on the one hand further helping his fundamental ideas to victory and on the other hand leading to a rich harvest of new facts.[35]

August Wassermann made a similar point about the heuristic value of scientific dissention, and pointed out that both sides of each of the arguments were stimulated to increased productivity,

> But we think of the opponents of the side-chain theory, among whom are found such outstanding and well-known investigators as Gruber, Bail, Bang and Forssmann, Bordet, and many others ... their prominent studies, undertaken as arguments against the side-chain theory, have actually worked to support it; on closer analysis they have contributed to a valuable enrichment of science.[36]

THE LIMITS OF PURE LOGIC

We saw in Chapters 5 through 7 that each time his results or ideas were challenged by apparently conflicting data, Ehrlich would first repeat the experiments to test the validity of the antagonist's results. He would then design additional experiments to establish the limits of applicability of the new phenomena. Finally, he would develop a further set of *ad hoc* assumptions that would serve to bring his earlier interpretations into line with those new observations that had seemed to cast doubt on them. Rarely would he abandon an earlier, published explanation in favor of an alternative, especially one proposed by a challenger.

Two examples, reviewed briefly, will testify to the extent to which Ehrlich could build layer upon layer of complication to adapt to new data. In the case of of the neutralization of diphtheria toxin by antitoxin, the sequence was roughly:

1. Such interactions must depend on firm organic chemical-like bonds, and therefore cannot be reversible.
2. As an irreversibile reaction, the neutralization must occur as an all-or-nothing event.
3. But the neutralization "curve" argues against a single discrete event. Therefore, there must be multiple components of differing affinities for antibody, interacting one after the other in a stepwise manner.[37]
4. This leads to the postulate, first of pro-, syn-, and epi-toxoids, and then of proto-, deutero-, and trito-toxins (in order of decreasing affinity).
5. Finally, since some components appear to be thermolabile and others thermostable, Ehrlich proposes α- and β-modifications of the several toxins.

Here is a congeries of components that could be fitted, in various proportions, to *any* neutralization curve.

The second example of the construction of a logical, albeit extremely complicated, schema to explain increasingly complex data involves the system of the
hemolysis of erythrocytes by antibody and complement. Again in brief outline:

1. The antitoxin molecule was originally credited with a single active site—
   that which binds it to toxin.
2. Hemolytic antibody only acts in conjunction with complement and therefore must also possess a separate complement-binding site.
3. But all receptors (even a complement receptor) must bind their partner molecules chemically, and thus specifically.
4. As each antibody-combining site (haptophore) is specific, so must each
   complementophore bind only its specific complement—therefore, there
   must exist a multiplicity of complements in any serum, one for each different anti-erythrocyte (hemolytic antibody) specificity.
5. But if, as Bordet showed, *any* antibody–antigen complex can fix all complements, it must be because each antibody has multiple complementophilic groups, a major one for *its* specific complement and many minor
   ones for all the other complements.
6. Finally, just as the toxophore group on diphtheria toxin can degrade to form
   a toxoid, so may the zymophore group on complement (that which dam-
   ages the red cell) degrade to form a "complementoid."

Now we have before us not only a multiplicity of complements, but in addition a
multipliicity of active receptor sites on the antibody molecule.

We shall not dwell here on Ehrlichs studies of anti-antibodies and anti-complements. Although the existence of these putative entities appeared just as logically derived from the data as the rest of Ehrlich's assortment of activities, he was
not alone in following up on this apparently reasonable interpretation. Many other
investigators at the time, including Metchnikoff, Bordet, and Besredka, failed to
realize that immunization with whole serum (be it an antiserum or merely an
active source of complement) would engender a host of complement-fixing antibodies against the many protein constituents of a serum.

HERR GEHEIMRATH EHRLICH

It is rare that any individual can be fitted accurately into a given mold that will
explain him or her fully and accurately, and this is certainly true of Paul Ehrlich.
We have, in this section, employed the rubric "Geheimrath" in part because
Ehrlich was awarded this title in fact, but in part also because the term has come
to imply a certain formal position and manner of action that fits Ehrlich to a certain extent. The term is not meant here to denigrate, but rather to describe the
position of the head of an institute or of a university department in 19th-century
Germany, a style quite common and accepted at the time.[38]

Ehrlich's Control of Research

From his earliest years as a medical student, and then later at the Charité and in Koch's Institute, Ehrlich had been a self-contained investigator, finding his own problems and doing most of the work himself. But always during these years (except for the period in 1890–1891 when his father-in-law supported him in a makeshift laboratory), he had worked in a large establishment subject to the whims of a Gerhardt or a Koch. Thus, when he was given his own Institute of Serum Research and Serum Testing in Steglitz in 1896, he could say *"Klein, aber mein!"*

The most notable feature of Ehrlich's activities once out on his own was that, no matter how large his establishment and how many different areas engaged, he was always in complete control at all levels. It was he who decided on the general area to be explored and also on the specific approaches to be undertaken. He would even plan individual experiments, often recommending to his associates the techniques to be used and even the amounts of reagent and numbers of test animals and controls to be employed. Part of the explanation for this intimate involvement was undoubtedly the fact that he appeared to know more about a given question than anyone else because he seemed to read everything published in the medical journals, even in areas of no apparent interest at the time. One has only to see the picture of Ehrlich's office (Plate 13), in which books, jornals, and reprints are stacked on the desk, the settee, the windowsill, and the floor, to appreciate the breadth of his reading (but if the office was cluttered, the mind was surely not). Thus, he would send notes (the famous *Blöke*) to his assistants suggesting that they read such-and-such an article in the German, French, Italian, or English literature. The other part of the explanation lay, of course, in a combination of an innately sharp insight and an overwhelming self-confidence.

Once he had attained the stature of a respected research leader, and had the direction of the Frankfurt Institute and then the Speyer Haus, Ehrlich's control over events could be followed day by day in the texts of his notes to fellow workers. He would request reports on experiments, suggest new ones, push people to finish work, send instructions on housekeeping matters and requests to order things, and write many notes (to others and to himself) on chemical reactions, often including structural diagrams and predictions of reaction products.[39] Thus:

> To Morgenroth: "Please do not forget tomorrow to change the supernatant (p. 233).
> To Shiga: "Please be most kind as to see me about … (p. 234).
> To Morgenroth: "Please look at a case of hemorrhagic diathesis by Bensanele in *Semaine Médicale,* 1903 p. 57 (p. 234).

Many of the notes start with such formalities as "I wanted to ask you…"; "I beg you to…"; "I should like also to inquire…"; or "Please, most amicably, show me tomorrow…"; and "I am most curious about…" He would often write to Shiga or Morgenroth "I would like you most amicably to show me all the animals tomorrow, so that…"

In a single 5-day period from January 21 to January 25, 1903, Ehrlich wrote 56 Blöke: to himself on the relationship of biological investigations to physical chemistry, on the concept of specificity, on chemical reactions, and so on; six to Sachs on immune hemolysis; nine to Sachs and Kyes on various toxins; one to secretary Marquardt as a reminder; 10 to Marx on anthrax and diphtheria immunizations; one to Shiga on trypanosomes; and so forth. One can almost determine the attendance records of the major players by whether or not Ehrlich sent them Blöke that day.

Thus, it is evident that Ehrlich ran a tight ship and did not provide significant independence to his collaborators, especially in those fields to which he was dedicated at the time. This is confirmed by Georg Schöne who, some 40 years later, commented on how it was to work for him.

> Paul Ehrlich was not a man whose principal interest it was to train his students for independent scientific work. *He worked and researched in his institute, and everyone had to subordinate himself* [his italics]. However, anyone who had occasion to work with him experienced a major advancement, and that especially in methodology. With Ehrlich, one learned to work.[40]

Another indication of Ehrlich's view of his research and his collaborators is that after 1893, of the 198 items in Ehrlich's bibliography, only three list another investigator as senior author. But two other observations mitigate this picture to an extent. First, once his interest in a certain area had given way to a new venture, those colleagues who had assisted in the earlier activities would continue those studies (e.g., immunology after 1901; tumor studies after 1905, etc.) and often publish independently (although often with the addendum that the work was performed "under the supervision/guidance of Geheimrath Ehrlich").

A second observation softens somewhat Schöne's indictment of Ehrlich's treatment of his collaborators. If, as Schöne claims, Ehrlich did not actively engage in the training of his associates for independent research, the result certainly was that a large number of them ended up as recognized independent investigators, much as modern-day postdoctoral fellows "learn the trade" from their mentors and then go off to practice independently. Thus, among others of Ehrlich's associates, Morgenroth became a professor in Berlin, Lazarus in Charlottenburg, Sachs in Frankfurt, Shiga and Hata in Tokyo, and Schöne himself in Greifswald.

A final word about Ehrlich's view of the manner in which research should be conducted. In the outline that Ehrlich prepared for the autobiographical note to be sent to Christian Herter in preparation for his American visit in 1904, Ehrlich wrote, "Work much, publish little: *pauca sed matura*. No preliminary communications. No guessing, exact measurements. Facts have always been all right with me."[41] This sentiment is strongly supported, first by the quantitative approach that he invariably employed in his work, and, second, by the quality of his bibliography. For a scientist who made substantial contributions to five different disciplines (histology, hematology, immunology, experimental oncology, and chemotherapy), a bibliography of 284 items, many of which are discussions at meetings of the work of others, is modest indeed.

Ehrlich's Relationship with Others

We have seen that if Ehrlich was a hard taskmaster, he was also invariably soft-spoken and polite with his coworkers and assistants. Indeed, contrary to the usual picture of a *Geheimrath*, Ehrlich seemed to have had no sense of self-importance. He gave himself only a small office in the institute, and preferred to wander the halls poking his head here and there, visiting colleagues rather than imperiously sending for them. When called on to explain an experiment or an idea, he would seize any nearby writing implement and write chemical equations or cartoon explanations on a host's napkin, a restaurant tablecloth, or even on his knees on the floor of his office. He apparently explained things in a very convoluted way, interspersing his sentences with *"Wissen Sie, verstehen Sie?"* [do you know, do you understand?]. As Henry Dale said, in remembering his own introduction to Ehrlich in 1904, "even if his own work and interests lay in a not distant field of medical research, the visitor was likely to find himself quite early out of his depth and to resign himself to submersion."[42]

Ehrlich's personal modesty is perhaps best illustrated by the following report by an out-of-town visitor.

> I went into the Royal Institute for Experimental Therapy to see the famous researcher. … Everything transpired differently than I had anticipated. … There was here no "Chef-zimmer," in the style of a General Director, with a diplomat's desk and clublike easy chairs, as is common today. There was nowhere a barrier for visitors; no anteroom protected the great man; there was no waiting room where one must wait at length before being admitted; rather, one dealt at once with Paul Ehrlich. On entering the corridor, I immediately bumped into the factotum Kadereit. No sooner did I mention my name, and that I was from Magdeburg, than he led me to Ehrlich with the words, "I believe that he is already waiting for you." And as I announced myself, I heard through the open door his clear voice, "Yes, fom Magdeburg, come right in," and I entered. … It was as if Ehrlich was in the middle of moving his residence. On the left was a sofa pressed down with tons of piled-up papers and books; then a bookcase that was unreachable because in front of it on chairs lay piles of similar publications at least 1 1/2 meters high. The window sill was similarly packed, and the right side of the room was likewise fully crammed. In the window corner was a small, simple desk of which only a corner remained clear, where the bottle of mineral water and the cigarbox stood, from which Ehrlich never parted. With a smiling, friendly glance, he laid aside his reading, and greeted me with his characteristic greeting, *'Tag ook,'* as though we had known one-another for a long time.[43]

He treated everyone thus, except for opponents like Max Gruber. When the great Emil Fischer came to the institute, after Ehrlich had received the Nobel Prize, the Prussian award of *Wirklicher Geheimrath* (right honorable Privy Councillor) with the title of *Excellenz,* and the rare Honorary Membership in the German Chemical Society, Ehrlich exclaimed, "Fancy *you* coming to see *me.*"[44] Ehrlich was invariably polite to his helpers and associates. He treated his secretary, Martha Marquardt, with consideration and respect, and she obviously adored him, as witnessed by her treatment of him in the biography she wrote.[45] Even his devoted attendant and factotum Wilhelm Kadereit was dealt with in kindly fashion as he served as doorkeeper, messenger, and provider of the ever-necessary cigars and mineral water. When, in 1902, Ehrlich learned from Almroth Wright of his forced departure from the Army Medical Establishment at Netley, he wrote letters to Wassermann, Bulloch, and several others, mentioning Wright's dispair and expressing his own dismay at this unfair treatment. In a letter to Wright,[46] Ehrlich offered his condolences, and asked whether he might write to Lord Lister to intercede on Wrights's behalf.

EHRLICH AT HOME

It is difficult to describe Paul Ehrlich, the private individual. One knows some-thing of the more superficial aspects of his personal life, but little about his activities outside the laboratory. There is little information about whether he attended the the-ater, the opera, or the symphony, or even whether he liked music (although he appar-ently always sang off-key). We know little about any underlying philosophical foun-dation, or whether he read broadly as was the fashion in the intellectual circles of the day. We only know that he read everything in experimental biology and medicine, and read detective stories for relaxation. He preferred Sherlock Holmes, and when Conan Doyle (a physician himself) learned of this, he sent Ehrlich a picture of him-self with a note expressing his appreciation of the scientist.

Ehrlich had enjoyed a classical education at the gymnasium in Strehlen, and ever after demonstrated a love of classical (especially Latin) sayings. He never missed an opportunity to use a Latin term or phrase, even to call down an oppo-nent like Gruber (e.g., *caput pigerrimum* = blockhead). In the same vein, in letters to his cousin Carl Weigert, he would address him as *Carole magne,* and Wasser-mann he called *Lieber Aquaticus,* among other jeux de mots.

Ehrlich was completely uninterested in politics, and apparently the one time that he went to vote in an election, Kadereit had to show him how it was done.[47] He took little interest in his religion, like many Jews of the German-Jewish "enlightenment," and did not observe the holy days. His secretary claims that it took her several years before she came to realize that Ehrlich was a Jew, but she suggests that he would not have dreamed of converting to forward his career[48] as did so many others, including Karl Landsteiner.[49] However, at the urging of Chaim Weizmann, Ehrlich did agree to serve on a committee to support the founding of the Hebrew University in Jerusalem.[50]

Ehrlich married Hedwig Pinkus in 1883, and they had two daughters, Stephanie in 1884 and Marianne in 1886. The daughters had five grandchildren between them, and Ehrlich doted on them. When they visited, he would take the older ones on nature walks, explaining various things to them. He would sing songs with them, recite poetry, and in the nursery make up fairy tales to amuse them, pretending that these extraordinary events had happened to him. But soon he would go off to his inner sanctum to work, not to be disturbed.[51]

He would work at home each morning, until Kadereit came with cigars, papers, and a carriage to take him to the institute. Almost every evening, he would take papers and journals home for further work. (He was always careful to carry them in a large envelope inscribed with his name and address, and the words, "Finder receives 10 marks"; more than once he had absentmindedly left these on the seat of his carriage.) Then, after dinner, he would excuse himself to return to his study to work and write out the next day's instructions to his colleagues on the colored Blöke, which Kadereit would copy the next morning and distribute. Even on Sunday, Kadereit would come with papers and off they would go to the institute. He would often arrive at work late and depart early, leaving much time, as he would say, for thinking on long walks, and for his detective stories. He would say often, "Quality over quantity."

Perhaps Ehrlich's dedication to his work is best characterized by Sir Henry Dale's depiction of Ehrlich, in his introduction to Marquardt's biography:

> I am sure that there are many who can confirm Miss Marquardt's memory and my own experience that, although Ehrlich had his occasional intervals of relaxation, in which he could show an almost childlike enjoyment of quiet fun and simple pleasures, his normal waking hours were filled withan extraordinary concentration of interest on his own scientific ideas and plans for research.[52]

POSTSCRIPT

The picture we have attempted to paint of Paul Ehrlich the scientist is quite obviously incomplete. The material available in the archives and in the reminiscences of friends and colleagues leaves gaps in the picture, perhaps never completely to be filled in. But this type of examination fails to do justice to the subject for another reason. Any detailed examination of the bits and pieces that make up the man and his science is like looking too closely at a pointillist painting; the colored marks on the canvas are too individually intrusive as to permit an appreciation of the entire figure to which they contribute. Only by standing apart, and viewing from a distance, may one begin to appreciate the overall value of the whole, which is the net product of a lifetime spent in science and in society.[53] From this perspective, Paul Ehrlich emerges, warts and all, as one of the great scientists of his time, and surely as one of the greatest polymaths of all biomedical science.

NOTES AND REFERENCES

1. Schöne, G., "Über Paul Ehrlichs Art, wissenschaftlich zu arbeiten," *Ärztliche Wochenschr.* 1:108, 1946, p. 110.
2. *Obsession:* 3. The persistent and unescapable influence of an idea. *Webster's New International Dictionary,* 2nd ed., 1922.
3. See, e.g., Wintrobe, M., *Hematology: the Blossoming of a Science,* Philadelphia, Lea & Febiger, 1985, especially p. 25.
4. A commemorative bronze plaque was struck to celebrate the First International Congress of Immunology, held in Washington, D.C. in 1971; It featured a portrait of Paul Ehrlich (see frontispiece).

5. Whereas Ehrlich's work in tumor transplantation was much discussed at the time; see Lewin, C., "Paul Ehrlichs Anteil an den Fortschritten der Krebsforschung," *Die Naturwiss.* 2:278, 1914. It is little remembered today, except for the eponymous *Ehrlich ascites tumor.*

6. See Parascandola J. and Jasensky, R., *Bull. Hist. Med.* 48:199, 1974, and Parascandola, J., *J. Hist. Med.* 36:19, 1981; also Loewe, H., "Paul Ehrlich, Schöpfer der Chemotherapie," in *Grosse Naturforscher,* vol. VIII, Stuttgart, Wissenschaftlicher Verlagsges., 1950; and Satter, H., *Paul Ehrlich, Begründer der Chemotherapie,* 2nd ed., Munich, Oldenbourg, 1963.

7. See Marquardt, M., *Paul Ehrlich,* London, William Heinemann, 1949, p. 15.

8. The landmark instructionist theory had been proposed by Breinl, F. and Haurowitz, F., *Z. Physiol. Chem.* 192:45, 1930. See also Mazumdar, P.M.H., in *Immunology, 1930–1980: Essays on the History of Immunology,* P.M.H. Mazumdar, ed., Toronto, Wall & Thompson, 1989, pp. 13–32. Haurowitz would rise once again in the history workshop at the VI International Congress of Immunology in 1986 to defend instruction theories.

9. See Bussard, A., "Darwinisme et Immunologie," *Bull. Soc. Franç. Philos.* 77:1, 1983.

10. Silverstein, A.M., *Cell. Immunol.* 48:208, 1979.

11. See, e.g., Silverstein, A.M., *A History of Immunology,* New York, Academic Press, 1989, pp. 99–104; Crist, E. and Tauber, A.I., *J. Hist. Biol.* 30:321, 1997.

12. See the discussions of the Ehrlich–Arrhenius dispute in Chapters 5.

13. Ehrlich, P., *Münch. med. Wochenschr.* 50:2295, 1903; *Collected Studies in Immunity* (C. Balduan, transl.), New York, Wiley, 1906, p. 514 ff.

14. Ehrlich, *Collected Studies,* note 13, p. viii.

15. These polemics and disputes can be found in Rockefeller Archives Center, Ehrlich Papers, 650 Eh 89 (henceforth RAC Ehrlich Papers), Box 3. There is a separate folder for each dispute.

16. Ehrlich's wrote so illegibly that the recipients of his *Blöke* often had to consult secretary Marquardt for translation, one of the few who could read his writing.

17. RAC Ehrlich Papers, Box 7, p. 248 (Beate Hirsch transl. box 55, folder 4).

18. RAC Ehrlich Papers, Box 8, p. 274 (Hirsch transl. box 55, folder 5).

19. RAC Ehrlich Papers, Box 8, p. 290 (Hirsch transl. box 55, folder 5).

20. RAC Ehrlich Papers, Box 9, p. 65 (Hirsch transl. box 55, folder 6).

21. RAC Ehrlich Papers, Box 9, p. 69 (Hirsch transl. box 55, folder 6).

22. RAC Ehrlich Papers, Box 9, p. 119 (Hirsch transl. box 55, folder 6).

23. RAC Ehrlich Papers, Box 9, p. 142 (Hirsch transl. box 55, folder 6).

24. RAC Ehrlich Papers, Box 9, p. 328 (Hirsch transl. box 55, folder 6).

25. RAC Ehrlich Papers, Box 5, p. 13 (Hirsch transl. Box 55, folder 2).

26. RAC Ehrlich Papers, Box 5, p. 26 (Hirsch transl. Box 55, folder 2).

27. RAC Ehrlich Papers, Box 5, p. 236 (Hirsch transl. Box 55, folder 2).

28. RAC Ehrlich Papers, Box 5, p. 344 (Hirsch transl. Box 55, folder 2).

29. RAC Ehrlich Papers, Box 6, p. 389 (Hirsch transl. Box 55, folder 3).

30. RAC Ehrlich Papers, Box 21, p. 151 (Hirsch transl. Box 55, folder 6).

31. RAC Ehrlich Papers, Box 23, p. 385.

32. RAC Ehrlich Papers, Box 23, pp. 8.

33. RAC Ehrlich Papers, Box 1, folder 8.

34. RAC Ehrlich Papers, Box 1, folder 8.

35. Gaffky G., in *Paul Ehrlich: Eine Darstellung seines wissenschaftichen Wirkens,* Jena, Gustav Fischer, 1914, p. 131 (henceforth *Ehrlich Festschrift*).

36. Wassermann, A., *Ehrlich Festschrift,* p. 148.

37. Here is another example, discussed earlier, of Ehrlich's preference for discontinuity as against continuity in physiological reactions; see note 15, Chapter 5.

38. One may compare the description of Ehrlich that follows with those of other more-or-less contemporary German laboratory chiefs discussed in Joseph Fruton's book, *Contrasts in Scientific Style: Research Groups in the Chemical and Biochemical Sciences,* Philadelphia, American Historical Society, 1990.

39. The following *Blöke* citations all come from Ehrlich's *"Zettelbuch IV,"* RAC Ehrlich Papers Box 10, for the period December 2, 1902 to November 5, 1903.
40. Schöne, note 1.
41. See Bäumler, E., *Paul Ehrlich, Scientist for Life,* New York, Holmes & Meier, 1984, p. 240.
42. Dale, H., in his introduction to Martha Marquardt's *Paul Ehrlich,* note 7, p. xvii.
43. Hans Schadewaldt, in his concluding talk at the opening of the Paul Ehrlich exhibit in Düsseldorf on January 28, 1981, quotes dermatologist A. Stühmer's description of a visit to Ehrlich in Frankfurt. Stühmer had sent this to Schadewaldt, who has kindly given me permission to reproduce it here.
44. Marquardt, *Paul Ehrlich,* note 7, p. 229.
45. Marquardt, *Paul Ehrlich,* note 7. Until her death in exile in London, she devoted herself to his memory, and encouraged Sir Henry Dale to become involved in sponsoring the preparation of *The Collected Papers of Paul Ehrlich.*
46. RAC Ehrlich Papers, Box 22, p. 329.
47. Marquardt, *Paul Ehrlich,* note 7, p. 160.
48. Marquardt, *Paul Ehrlich,* note 7, p. 160.
49. See Speiser, P. and Smekal, F.G., *Karl Landsteiner: The Discoverer of Blood Groups and a Pioneer in the Field of Immunology* (R. Rickett transl.), Vienna, Brüder Hollinek, 1975.
50. Bäumler (in *Paul Ehrlich,* note 41, pp. 212–214) tells the amusing story of Weizmann's visit to solicit Ehrlich's support of the Hebrew University, made at the urging of the Baron de Rothschild whose financial aid would be critical. Weizmann, hardly expecting more than five minutes with the great man, was recognized by Ehrlich as a "fellow" chemist and subjected for more than an hour to his typical energetic, if difficult, lecture. When at last Weizmann could get a word in edgewise to explain his mission, Ehrlich took him home for dinner, and finally agreed to serve. See Weizmann, C., *Trial and Error,* New York, Harper, 1949. Ehrlich later wrote to Baron de Rothschild urging his support of the university, and referred therein to "my good friend Weizmann" (RAC Ehrlich Papers, Box 1, folder 42).
51. The foregoing is based on personal conversations (in 1995) with Günther Schwerin [1910–1997], Ehrlich's grandson and younger son of daughter Stephanie, and confirmed in large part in Marquardt's *Paul Ehrlich,* note 7 and Bäumler's *Paul Ehrlich,* note 41.
52. Dale, H., in Marquardt's *Paul Ehrlich,* note 7, p. xvii.
53. This is one of the problems with the modern vogue of historical deconstruction, so popular among many contemporary historians of science and medicine. The result of such fine sifting of methods, data, and interpretations is to lose completely the view of the individual as a whole. From such an approach, which too often overemphasizes the negatives, comes the facile conclusion that "there are no more heroes."

PAUL EHRLICH'S HONORS[1]

TITLES GRANTED

1891 Named *Ausserordentlicher Professor* (Adjunct Professor), University of Berlin

1896 Director, *Institut für Serumforschung und Serumprüfung* (Institute for Serum Research and Testing), Steglitz, Berlin

1897 Named *Geheimer Medizinalrath* (Medical Privy Councillor)

1899 Director, *Institut für Experimentelle Therapie* (Institute for Experimental Therapy), Frankfurt am Main

1904 Named Honorary Professor, University of Göttingen

1906 Director, Georg Speyer Haus (for chemotherapy research)

1907 Named *Geheimer Obermedizinalrath* (Medical High Privy Councillor)

1911 Named *Wirklicher Geheimrath* ('Real' Privy Councillor)[2] with the title *Excellenz*

1914 Named *Ordentlicher Professor,* University of Frankfurt

PRIZES, MEDALS, AND DISTINGUISHED LECTURESHIPS

1887 *Tiedemann Prize* of the Senckenburg Naturforschende Gesellschaft, Frankfurt

1900 *Croonian Lecture,* The Royal Society, London

1904 *Herter Lectures,* Johns Hopkins University, Baltimore

1906 *Prize of Honor,* XV International Congress of Medicine, Lisbon

---

1. Most of the material described here is recorded in the Paul Ehrlich Collection at the Rockefeller Archives Center, 650 Eh89, Box 2, folders 6–20. See also Marquardt, M., *Paul Ehrlich*, London, Heinemann, 1949, pp. 251–255.

2. The two earlier titles of *Geheimer Rath* are honorifics; the adjective *Wirklicher* is both honorific and intended to imply an actual duty as counselor. Perhaps the best translation would be "Right Honorable Privy Councillor.

1907 *Harben Lecture,* Royal Institute of Public Health, London

1908 *Nobel Prize* for Medicine or Physiology (with Elie Metchnikoff)

1911 *Liebig Médaille,* Society of German Chemists

1914 *Cameron Prize,* Edinburg

ORDERS AWARDED

Bavaria	*Maximilian Order*
Denmark	*Commander Cross, Dannebrog Order, 2nd Degree*
Japan	*Order of the Rising Sun, 3rd Degree*
Norway	*Commander Cross, Royal Norwegian St. Olaf Order, 2nd Degree*
Palatinate	*Cavalier Cross, Order of Berthold I of Zähringen*
Prussia	*Order of the Crown, 2nd Degree*
	Order of the Red Eagle, 2nd Degree
Romania	*Cross for Sanitary Merit, 1st Degree*
Russia	*Order Of St. Anne, 1st Degree, with Diamonds, Star, and Cross*
Serbia	*Great Cross of the Order of St. Sava*
Spain	*Great Cross, Order of Alfonso XII, with Star and Cross*
Venezuela	*Great Cross of the Bust of Bolivar, 2nd Degree*

HONORARY DEGREES

1904 LL.D., University of Chicago

1907 D.C.L., Oxford University

1911 Dr. Phil., University of Athens

1912 Dr. Med., University of Breslau

HONORARY MEMBERSHIPS

1900 Balneological Society, Berlin
Royal Danish Society of Sciences, Copenhagen

1902 International Society for the Fight against Tuberculosis, Berlin

1903 Silesian Society for Home Culture, Breslau
Royal Academy of Medicine, Turin

1904 Royal Academy of Science, Bologna
Society for Internal Medicine, Vienna
Imperial and Royal Society of Physicians, Vienna
New York Academy of Medicine, New York

Royal Society of Sciences, Göttingen
National Academy of Science, Washington, D.C.
Societas Therapeutical Mosquana, Moscow

1905   Académie de Médicine, Paris
       Medical Society, Budapest

1906   Medical Society of Finland, Helsingfors
       Society of Physicians, Munich
       Société de Biologie, Paris

1907   Pathological Society of Great Britain and Ireland, London
       Society of Tropical Medicine and Hygiene, London
       Royal Academy dei Lincei, Rome
       Royal Institute of Public Health, London
       Medical Society of Berlin

1908   Société de Pathologie Exotique, Paris
       Physical-Medical Society, Erlangen
       Society for the Knowledge of Nature and Medical Treatment, Dresden
       Swedish Medical Society, Stockholm
       Physical Society, Frankfurt

1909   Medical Society, St. Petersburg

1910   Microbiological Society, St. Petersburg
       The Royal Society, London
       Imperial Medical Society of the Caucasus
       Royal Swedish Academy of Sciences, Stockholm
       German Society for Tropical Medicine, Hamburg
       Society of Physicians, Odessa
       Khedivial Society of Medicine, Cairo
       Medical Society of Yekaterinoslav
       Vienna Dermatological Society
       Medical Society of Serbia, Belgrade
       Physical-Medical Society of Saratov

1911   Union of St. Petersburg Physicians
       Imperial Society of Medicine, Constantinople
       Royal Society of Sciences, Uppsala
       Academia Romana, Bucharest
       Union of Physicians, Smolensk
       Microbiological Society, Delft
       Royal Medical Society, Edinburg
       Royal Academy of Medicine, Brussels
       Imperial institute for Experimental Therapy, St. Petersburg

1912   Physiological Society of London
       Society of Internal Medicine, Berlin
       Cancer Research Society of the Palatinate, Heidelberg

Kharkov Veterinary Institute
Brazilian Dermatological Society, Rio de Janeiro
National Academy of Venezuela, Caracas
Royal Society of Medicine and Natural Science, Brussels
Dermatological Society of Odessa
Medical Society of Athens

1913   Society for Natural Sciences, Braunschweig
German Chemical Society, Berlin
Union of Physicians, Archangel
Society of Physicians, Odessa
Society of German Physicians of Mental Diseases, Berlin
Medical Society of Orel
Society of Veterinary Doctors, Kazan
Harveian Society of London
Society of Biology, Paris
Italian Society of Dermatologists, Rome

1914   Medical-Surgical Society of Bologna
Society of Specialists for Children, Moscow
Norwegian Society of Natural Sciences, Christiana
Society of Jewish Physicians of the Ottoman Empire, Constantinople

1915   Pharmaceutical Society, Berlin

PAUL EHRLICH'S
SCIENTIFIC
BIBLIOGRAPHY

This bibliography is based primarily on one prepared by Dr. Fred Himmelweit around 1960 that was intended for inclusion in volume IV of *The Collected Papers of Paul Ehrlich;* for reasons unknown, that volume was never published. The bibliography, annotated in Himmelweit's hand, was found in February 2000 among the Henry Dale papers in the Archives of the Royal Society of London (No. 93HD 64.5), and is utilized here with the permission of the Royal Society. It represents Himmelweit's revision and update of the Ehrlich bibliography compiled by Hans Sachs for *Paul Ehrlich: Eine Darstellung seines wissenschaftlichen Wirkens* (Jena, Gustav Fischer, 1914) a Festschrift prepared in honor of Ehrlich's 60th birthday. (The Sachs bibliography also contains references to the independently-published works by Ehrlich's scientific associates.) Several additions to this list were taken from the Ehrlich bibliography published by Ernst Bäumler in his *Paul Ehrlich: Scientist for Life* (New York, Holmes & Meier, 1984); other additions and title translations have been made by the present author.

Many of the immunological papers of Paul Ehrlich were published in *Gesammelte Arbeiten zur Immunitätsforschung* (Berlin, Hirschwald, 1904); abbreviated here as *Gesammelte Arbeiten.* An English translation of the German edition, entitled *Collected Studies on Immunity,* was edited by C. Bolduan (New York, Wiley; London, Chapman and Hall, 1906), and is abbreviated here as *Collected Studies.* Later Himmelweit, under the aegis of Sir Henry Dale, compiled the three volumes of *The Collected Papers of Paul Ehrlich:* I. Histology, Biochemistry, and Pathology; II. Immunology and Cancer Research: III. Chemotherapy (London, Pergamon, 1956–1960). These contain most of the original publications plus English translations of those then considered the most important. They are abbreviated here as *Collected Papers,* with the appropriate volume number.[1]

The inclusion of a city and date in parentheses indicates that an oral presentation was made before the society cited.

---

1. For a description of the search for an explanation of why volume IV was never published, see Silverstein, A. M., *Bull. Hist. Med.* 75 No. 3, 2001.

1877

1. Beiträge zur Kenntnis der Anilinfärbung und ihrer Verwendung in der mikroskopischen Technik [Contributions to the knowledge of aniline staining and its application to microscopic technic]. *Arch. mikr. Anat.* 13:263–277, 1877; *Collected Papers* vol. I, pp. 19–28.

1878

2. Beiträge zur Theorie und Praxis der histologischen Färbung [Contributions to the theory and practice of histological staining]. Inaugural-Dissertation der Medizinischen Fakultät der Universität Leipzig, vorgelegt am 17 Juni, 1878 (then unpublished); *Collected Papers* vol. I, pp. 29–64.

2a. Contributions to the theory and practice of histological staining (Translation of No. 2); *Collected Papers* vol. I, pp. 65–98.

1879

3. Beiträge zur Kenntnis der granulierten Bindegewebszellen und der eosinophilen Leucocyten [Contributions to the knowledge of granulated connective tissue cells and of eosinophilic leukocytes]. Verh. Phys. Ges. (Berlin 17.1.1879); *Arch. Anat. Physiol.* (Physiol. Abt.) pp. 166–169, 1879; *Collected Papers* vol. I, pp. 114–116.

4. Ueber die spezifischen Granulationen des Blutes [On the specific granulations of the blood]. Verh. Phys. Ges. (Berlin 16.5.1879); *Arch. Anat. Physiol.* (Physiol. Abt.) pp. 571–579; *Collected Papers* vol. I, pp. 117–123.

1880

5. Ueber syphilitische Herzinfarkte [On syphilitic myocardial infarcts]. *Z. klin. Med.* 1:378–381, 1880; *Collected Papers* vol. I, pp. 99–102.

6. Methodologische Beiträge zur Physiologie und Pathologie der verschiedenen Formen der Leukozyten [Methodological contributions to the physiology and pathology of various forms of leukocytes]. *Z. klin. Med.* 1:553–560, 1880; *Collected Papers* vol. I, pp. 124–129.

7. Beobachtungen über einen Fall von perniziöser, progressiver Anämie mit Sarcombildung: Beiträge zur Lehre von der acuten Herzinsufficienz [Observations on a case of progressive pernicious anemia with sarcoma formation: Contributions to the study of acute cardiac insufficiency]. *Charité-Ann.* 5:189–205, 1880; *Collected Papers* vol. I, pp. 130–134.

8. Über Regeneration und Degeneration rother Blutscheiben bei Anämien [On regeneration and degeneration of red blood corpuscles in anemia patients]. Ges. Charité-Aerzte (Berlin 10.6.1880); *Berl. klin. Wochenschr.* 28:405, 1880; *Collected Papers* vol. I, p. 135.

9. Über einige Beobachtungen am anämischen Blut [On some observations on anemic blood]. Ges. Charité-Aerzte (Berlin 9.12.1880); *Berl. klin. Wochenschr.* 18:43, 1880; *Collected Papers* vol. I, pp. 136–137.

1881

10. Vorstellung eines Falles von Echinococcus hepatis [Presentation of a case of echinococcus of the liver]. Verh. Charité-Aerzte (Berlin 27.1.1881); *Berl. klin. Wochenschr.* 18:202, 1881 (title only).

11. Ueber provocirte Fluorescenzerscheinungen am Auge [On the induced appearance of fluorescence in the eye]. Ges. Charité-Aerzte (Berlin 10.3.1881); *Deutsch. med. Wochenschr.* 8:21–22, 35–37, 54–55, 1882; *Collected Papers* vol. I, pp. 344–353.

12. Über paroxysmale Hämoglobinurie [On paroxysmal hemoglobinuria]. Verh. Ver. Inn. Med. (Berlin 21.3.1881); *Deutsch. med. Wochenschr.* 7:224–225, 1881; *Z. klin. Med.* 3:383, 1881; *Collected Papers* vol. I, pp. 138–140.

13. Über Befunde am Tinctionspräparat eines Falles von lymphatischer Leukämie [On the findings in a stained preparation from a case of lymphatic leukemia]. Verh. Ver. Inn. Med. (Berlin 16.5.1881); 1:52–53, 1882; *Deutsch. med. Wochenschr.* 7:341, 1881; *Z. klin. Med.* 3:407–408, 1881.

14. Ueber carcinöse Pleuritis [On carcinomatous pleuritis]. Verh. Charité-Aerzte (Berlin 16.6.1881); *Berl. klin. Wochenschr.* 18:605, 1881.

15. Ueber das Methylenblau und seine klinisch-bakterioskopische Verwertung [On methylene blue and its clinico-bacterioscopic application]. *Z. klin. Med.* 2:710–713, 1881; *Collected Papers* vol. I, pp. 287–289.

16. Zur Genese der Herzinfarcte [On the genesis of cardiac infarcts]. *Zbl. med. Wiss.* 19:753–756, 1881; *Collected Papers* vol. I, pp. 354–356.

1882

17. Beiträge zur Aetiologie und Histologie pleuritischer Exsudate: I. Ueber die Pleuritis im Wochenbett, etc; II. Zur Diagnostik der carcinomatösen Pleuritis [Contributions to the etiology and histology of pleuritic exudates: I. On pleuritis in puerperium, etc.; II. On the diagnosis of carcinomatous pleuritis]. *Charité-Ann.* 7:199–230, 1882; *Collected Papers* vol. I, pp. 290–310.

18. Ueber einen Fall von Phosphorvergiftung mit symmetrischer Gangrena pedum [On a case of phosphorus poisoning with symmetrical gangrene of the feet]. *Charité-Ann.* 7:231–236, 1882; *Collected Papers* vol. I, pp. 526–529.

19. Über eine neue Harnreaction [On a new urine reaction]. Ges. Charité-Aerzte (Berlin 13.4.1882); *Berl. klin. Wochenschr.* 20:13, 1882.

20. Ueber eine neue Harnprobe [On a new urine test]. *Z. klin. Med.* 5:285–288, 1882 (cf. # 19); *Collected Papers* vol. I, pp. 619–629.

21. Über eine neue Methode der Färbung von Tuberkelbacillen [On a new method for the staining of tubercle bacilli]. Ges. Charité-Aerzte (Berlin 27.4.1882); *Berl. klin. Wochenschr.* 20:13, 1882.

22. Modification der von Koch angegebenen Methode der Färbung von Tuberkelbacillen [Modification of Koch's method for the staining of tubercle bacilli]. Verh. Ver. Inn. Med. (Berlin 1.5.1882); 2:31–34, 1882 (discussion, 34–35); *Z. klin. Med.* 5:307–309, 1882; *Deutsch. med. Wochenschr.* 8:269–270, 1882 (discussion, 365); *Collected Papers* vol. I, pp. 311–313.

23. Discussion of "über den plötzlichen Tod und das Coma der Diabetiker" [On the sudden death and coma of diabetics] by F. Th. Frerichs. Verh. Ver. Inn. Med. (Berlin 3.7.1882); 2:56–58, 74, 76, 1883.

24. Discussion of demonstration, "Mikrokokken bei einem Fall von akutem Gelenkrheumatismus" [Micrococci in a case of acute rheumatoid arthritis] by E. Leyden. Verh. Ver. Inn. Med. (Berlin 17.7.1882); 2:82–83, 84, 1883.

25. Brieger, L. and Ehrlich, Ueber das Auftreten des malignen Oedems bei Typhus abdominalis [On the appearance of malignent edema in abdominal typhus]. *Berl. klin. Wochenschr.* 19:661–665, 1882; *Deutsch. med. Wochenschr.* 8:604–606, 1882 (Abstract); *Collected Papers* vol. I, pp. 314–321.

26. Über Resultate mit Sulfanilsäure [On results with sulfanilic acid]. Ges. Charité-Aerzte (Berlin, 2.11.1882); *Berl. klin. Wochenschr.* 20:135, 1882.

1883

27. Ueber das Vorkommen von Glykogen im diabetischen und im normalen Organismus [On the occurrence of glycogen in diabetic and normal organisms]. Appendix 1 in F. Th. Frerichs: Ueber den plötzlichen Tod und über das Coma bei Diabetes [On sudden death and coma in diabetes]. *Z. klin. Med.* 6:3–53, 1883; loc. cit. 33–46; *Collected Papers* vol. I, pp. 103–112.

28. Über die gegen R. Kochs Entdeckung der Tuberkelbacillen neuerlichst hervorgetretenen Einwände [On the most recent objections advanced against R. Koch's discovery of tubercle bacilli]. Verh. Ver. Inn. Med. (Berlin, 5.3.1883); 2:207–217, 1883 (incl. discussion); *Z. klin. Med.* 6:574–577, 1883; *Deutsch. med. Wochenschr.* 9:159–162, 1883; *Collected Papers* vol. I, pp. 322–329.

29. Ueber eine neue Harnprobe [On a new urine test]. *Charité-Ann.* 8:140–166, 1883.

30. Einige Worte über die Diazoreaktion [Some comments on the diazoreaction]. *Deutsch. med. Wochenschr.* 9:549–552, 1883.

31. Sulfodiazobenzol, ein Reagens auf Bilirubin [Sulfodiazobenzene, a reagent for bilirubin]. *Zbl. klin. Med.* 4:721–723, 1883; *Collected Papers* vol. I, pp. 630–631.

32. Demonstration eines leukämischen Blutpräparates [Demonstration of a leukemic blood preparation]. Verh. Ver. Inn. Med. (Berlin, 5.11.1883); 3:133–134, 1884; *Deutsch. med. Wochenschr.* 9:670, 1883; *Collected Papers* vol. I, pp. 141–142.

1884

33. Zur Kenntnis des acuten Milztumors [On the knowledge of acute splenic tumor]. *Charité-Ann.* 9:107–114, 1884 *Collected Papers* vol. I, pp. 143–147.

34. Ehrlich and L. Brieger. Ueber die Ausschaltung des Lendenmarkgrau [On the loss of lumbar medullary gray matter]. *Z. klin. Med.* 7(Suppl.):155–164, 1884; *Collected Papers* vol. I, pp. 357–363.

35. Discussion of "Haemorrhagische-Diathese bei linealer Leukämie" [Hemmorhagic diathesis in leukemia] by S.A. Zwicke. Verh. Charité-Aerzte (Berlin, 1.5.1884); 21:414–415, 1884.

36. Ueber die Sulfodiazobenzol Reaktion [On the sulfodiazobenzene reaction]. Verh. Ver. Inn. Med. (Berlin, 16.6.1884); 4:47–61, 1885; *Deutsch. med. Wochenschr.* 10:419–422, 1884 [discussion p. 430]; *Collected Papers* vol. I, pp. 632–642.

37. Ueber das Sauerstoffbedürfnis im Organismus [On the oxygen requirement in the organism]. Verh. Charité-Aerzte (Berlin, 18.12.1884); *Berl. klin. Wochenschr.* 22:359, 1885 (title only).

1885

38. Discussion of demonstration "Einige Fälle von Chorea" [Several cases of chorea] by E. Henoch. Verh. Charité-Aerzte (Berlin, 8.1.1885). *Berl. klin. Wochenschr.* 22:500, 1885.

39. Discussion of demonstration "Ein auf operativem Wege geheilter Fall von Ileus" [A case of ileus cured by operative means] by A. Köhler. Verh. Charité-Aerzte (Berlin, 8.1.1885); *Berl. klin. Wochenschr.* 22:500, 501, 1885.

40. Das Sauerstoffbedürfnis des Organismus: eine Farbenanalytische Studie [The requirement of the organism for oxygen: a dye-analytical study]. Berlin, Hirschwald, 1885, 167pp.; *Collected Papers* vol. I, pp. 364–432.

40a. The requirement of the organism for oxygen: a dye-analytical study (Translation of No. 40); *Collected Papers* vol. I, pp. 433–496.

41. Zur biologischen Verwertung des Methylenblau [On the biological application of methylene blue. *Zbl. med. Wiss.* 23:113–117, 1885; *Collected Papers* vol. I, pp. 497–499.

42. Antikritische Bemerkungen über Drüsenfunctionen [Countercritical observations on the function of glands]. *Zbl. med. Wiss.* 23:161–165, 1885.

43. Ueber Wesen und Behandlung des Jodismus [On the nature and treatment of iodine poisoning]. *Charité-Ann.* 10:129–135, 1885; *Collected Papers* vol. I, pp. 530–534.

44. Zur Physiologie und Pathologie der Blutscheiben: A. Ueber die Functionen des Discoplasmas. B. Ueber Blutkörperchengifte nebst Betrachtungen über paroxystische Hämoglobinurie [On the physiology and pathology of blood cells: A. On the functions of erythrocyte cytoplasm; B. On blood cell poisons together with considerations on paroxysmal hemoglobinuria]. *Charité-Ann.* 10:136–146, 1885; 148–154.

45. Demonstration eines Krankes mit tuberculösem Lippengeschwür [Demonstration of a patient with tuberculous lip ulcer]. Ges. Charité-Aerzte (Berlin 30.4.1885); *Berl. klin. Wochenschr.* 22:665, 1885.

46. Book Review "De la Phthisie Bacillaire des Poumons" [On bacillary phthisis of the lungs] by Prof. G. Sée, Paris, Delahaye et Lacrosnier, *Z. klin. Med.* 9:498–500, 1885.

47. Ehrlich and B. Laquer, Ueber continuirliche Thallinzuführung und deren Wirkung beim Abdominaltyphus [On continuous administration of thallin and its effect on abdominal typhus]. Ges. Charité-Aerzte (Berlin, 19.11.1885); *Berl. klin. Wochenschr.* 22:837–841, 855–862, 1885; [French transl., Paris, Davy, 1885, 23 pp.; English transl. New York, 1886, 24pp.]; *Collected Papers* vol. I, pp. 535–541.

48. Reply to G. Gerhardt, discussion on tubercle bacilli in the sputum in early phthisis. Verh. Charité-Aerzte (Berlin 19.11.1885); *Berl. klin. Wochenschr.* 23:163, 1885.

49. Ueber die Methylenblaureaction der lebenden Nervensubstanz [On the methylene blue reaction of living nerve substance]. Verh. Ver. Inn. Med. (Berlin, 21.12.1885); 5:170–181, 1885; *Deutsch. med. Wochenschr.* 12:49–52, 1886; *Biol. Zbl.* 6:214–224, 1886/87; [French transl. *Gaz. Méd. Paris* 3:64–75, 1886; *Collected Papers* vol. I, pp. 500–508.

1886

50. Discussion of demonstration "Ueber Anstrengung des Herzens" [On the exertion of the heart] by O. Fräntzel. Verh. Charité-Aerzte (Berlin, 28.1.1886); *Berl. klin. Wochenschr.* 23:505, 1886.

51. Die von mir herrührende Hämatoxylinlösung [On my original hematoxylin solution]. (Reply to an editorial query). *Z. wiss. Mikr.* 3:150, 1886; *Collected Papers* vol. I, p. 113.

52. Beiträge zur Theorie der Bacillenfärbung [Contributions to the theory of the staining of bacilli]. *Charité-Ann.* 11:123–138, 1886; reprinted, Berlin, Hirschwald, 17 pp.; *Collected Papers* vol. I, pp. 330–339.

53. Nachträgliche Bemerkungen zur Diazoreaction: 1. Ueber den Bilirubinnachweis; 2. Ueber das primäre Eigelb [Supplementary remarks on the diazoreaction: 1. On the evidence of bilirubin; 2. On primary vitellin]. *Charité-Ann.* 11:139–142, 1886; *Collected Papers* vol. I, pp. 643–645.

54. Experimentelles und Klinisches über Thallin [Experimental and clinical items about thallin]. Verh. Ver. Inn. Med. (Berlin, 15.11.1886). 6:138–151, 151–155, 1887; *Deutsch. med. Wochenschr.* 12:849–851, 889–891; 899–900, 1886; *Collected Papers* vol. I, pp. 542–551.

1887

55. Schädliche Wirkung grosser Thallindosen [Harmful effects of large doses of thallin]. *Therap. Monatsh.* 1:53–54, 1887.

56. Zur therapeutischen Bedeutung der substituirenden Schwefelsäuregruppe [On the therapeutic meaning of substituted sulfonic acid groups]. *Therap. Monatsh.* 1:88–90, 1887; *Collected Papers* vol. I, pp. 552–554.

57. Ueber Pleuritis [On pleuritis]. Ges. Charité-Aerzte (Berlin, 24.2.1887).; *Berl. klin. Wochenschr.* 24:579–580, 1887.

58. Ueber die Körnchen in den Blutkörperchen [On the granules in blood cells]. Ges. Charité-Aerzte (Berlin, 21.4.1887). *Berl. klin. Wochenschr.* 24:657, 1887 (title only); *Collected Papers* vol. I, pp. 340–341.

59. Ueber die Bedeutung der neutrophilen Körnung [On the meaning of neutrophilic granules]. *Charité-Ann.* 12:288–295, 1887; *Collected Papers* vol. I, pp. 155–159.

60. Discussion of "Ueber eine indigobildende Substanz in eine Pleuraexsudat" [On an indigo-forming substance in a pleural exsudate] by P. Guttmann. Verh. Ver. Inn. Med. (Berlin, 5.12.1887); 7:251–254, 1888.

1888

61. Discussion of "Ueber Empyem" [On empyema] by A. Fränkel. Verh. Charité-Aerzte (Berlin, 5.1.1888); *Berl. klin. Wochenschr.* 25:408, 1888; *Collected Papers* vol. I, pp. 342–343.

62. Ueber einen Fall von Anämie mit Bemerkungen über regenerative Veränderungen des Knochenmarks [On a case of anemia with observations on

regenerative changes in the bone marrow]. *Charité-Ann.* 13:300–309, 1888; *Collected Papers* vol. I, pp. 160–165.

63. Discussion of "Ueber Lebercirrhose" [On cirrhosis of the liver] by E. Henoch. (Berlin, 16.2.1888); *Berl. klin. Wochenschr.* 25:635, 1888.

64. Experimentell-pharmakologische Untersuchungen [Experimental-pharmacological investigations]. Verh. Charité-Aerzte (Berlin, 1.3.1888); *Berl. klin. Wochenschr.* 25:675, 1888 (title only).

65. Discussion of "Zur Aetiologie der perniciösen Anämic" [On the etiology of pernicious anemia] by F. Müller. Ges. Charité-Aerzte (Berlin, 14.6.1888); *Berl. klin. Wochenschr.* 26:17, 1899.

1890

66. Ehrlich and A. Leppmann. Ueber schmerzstillende Wirkung des Methylenblau [On the analgesic effect of methylene blue]. *Deutsch. med. Wochenschr.* 16:493–494, 1890; *Collected Papers* vol. I, pp. 555–558.

67. Studien in der Cocainreihe [Studies of cocain analogs]. *Deutsch. med. Wochenschr.* 16:717–719, 1890; *Collected Papers* vol. I, pp. 559–566.

1891

68. Discussion of demonstration "Ein nach Koch behandelter Fall von Tuberculose" [A case of tuberculosis treated according to Koch] by H. Senator. (Berlin, 22.1.1891); *Berl. klin. Wochenschr.* 28:165–167, 180–181, 1891.

69. Guttmann, P. and Ehrlich, Entgegnung auf die Mittheilung über Tuberkelbacillen im Blut nach Kochschen Injectionen [Response to the report on tubercle bacilli in the blood following Koch-type injections]. *Deutsch. med. Wochenschr.* 17:251, 1891.

70. Guttmann, P. and Ehrlich, über Anfangsbehandlung der Lungen- und Kehlkopftuberkulose mit Kochschem Tuberkulin [On the initial treatment of lung and laryngeal tuberculosis with Koch's tuberculin]. *Deutsch. med. Wochenschr.* 17:373, 1891; *Münch. med. Wochenschr.* 38:196, 1891 (abstract only).

71. Guttmann, P. and Ehrlich, Die Wirksamkeit kleiner Tuberkulindosen gegen Lungenschwindsucht [The efficacy of small doses of tuberculin against phthisis]. *Deutsch. med. Wochenschr.* 17:793, 1891; *Collected Papers* vol. II, pp. 7–12.

72. On Ricin and Abrin, in a general discussion on immunity. 7th Int. Congr. Hygiene, Sect. II Bacteriol. (London, 1891). 2:177, 1891.

73. Ueber neuere Erfahrungen in der Behandlung der Tuberkulose nach Koch, insbesondere der Lungenschwindsucht [On the newer experiences in the treatment of tuberculosis according to Koch, especially of phthisis]. 7th Int. Congr. Hygiene, Sect. II, Bacteriol. (London, 1891). 2:211–220; *Lancet* 2:919–920, 1891 (abstract); *Münch. med. Wochenschr.* 38:691, 1891 (abstract); *Collected Papers* vol. II, pp. 13–20.

74. Guttmann, P. and Ehrlich. Ueber die Wirkung des Methylenblau bei Malaria [On the action of methylene blue in malaria]. *Berl. klin. Wochenschr.* 28:953–956, 1891; *Collected Papers* vol. III, pp. 9–14.

74a. On the action of methylene blue in malaria (Translation of No. 74); *Collected Papers* vol. III, pp. 15–20.

75. Experimentelle Untersuchungen über Immunität. I. über Ricin [Experimental investigations on immunity. I. On ricin]. *Deutsch. med. Wochenschr.* 17:976–979, 1891; *Collected Papers* vol. II, pp. 21–26.

76. Experimentelle Untersuchungen über Immunität. II. über Abrin [Experimental investigations on immunity. II. On abrin]. *Deutsch. med. Wochenschr.* 17:1218–1219, 1891; *Collected Papers* vol. II, pp. 27–30.

77. Zur Geschichte der Granula [On the history of granules]. (Included in No. 78, below, as paper XII, pp. 134–137); *Collected Papers* vol. I, pp. 166–168.

78. Farbenanalytische Untersuchungen zur Histologie und Klinik des Blutes [Dye-analytical investigations on the histology and clinic of the blood]. Berlin: Hirschwald, 1891, iv + 137 pp. (Comprises a foreword, three contributions by other authors, and Nos. 3, 4, 6, 8, 9, 12, 44, 59, 62, and 77 above.)

1892

79. Ueber Immunität durch Vererbung und Säugung [On Immunity through heredity and suckling]. *Z. Hyg. Infektkr.* 12, 183–203, 1892; *Collected Papers* vol. II, pp. 31–44.

80. Brieger, L. and Ehrlich. Ueber die Uebertragung von Immunität durch Milch [On the transfer of immunity by milk]. *Deutsch. med. Wochenschr.* 18:393–394, 1892; *Collected Papers* vol. II, pp. 45–47.

81. Bemerkungen über die Immunität durch Vererbung und Säugung. [Observations on immunity by heredity and suckling]. *Deutsch. med. Wochenschr.* 18:511, 1892.

82. Über schwere anämische Zustande [On severe anemic conditions]. Verh. 11 Deutsch. Kongr. Inn. Med. (Leipzig, 1892). 11:33–52, 1892; discussion, loc. cit., 11:63–64, 1892; *Collected Papers* vol. I, pp. 169–180.

1893

83. Brieger, L. and Ehrlich, Beiträge zur Kenntniss der Milch immunisierte Tiere [Contributions to the knowledge of the milk of immunized animals]. *Z. Hyg. Infektkr* 13:336–346, 1893; *Collected Papers* vol. II, pp. 48–55.

84. Ehrlich and G. Cohn, Die Einwirkung von Säurechloriden auf Nitrosodimethylanilin [The influence of acyl chlorides on nitrosodimethylaniline]. *Ber. deutsch. chem. Ges.* 26:1756–1757, 1893; *Collected Papers* vol. I, pp. 509–510.

85. Ueber Farbstoffreactionen (Neutralroth) [On staining reactions (neutral red)]. Verh. Ver. Inn. Med. (Berlin 18.12.1893). 13:183, 1894; *Allg. med. Zentralztg* 2:20, 1894 (abstract); *Berl. klin. Wochenschr.* 31:500, 1894; *Z. wiss. Mikr.* 11:250, 1894; *Collected Papers* vol. I, p. 511.

86. Constitution, Vertheilung, und Wirkung chemischer Koerper: aeltere und neuere Arbeiten [The constitution, distribution, and activity of chemical bodies: older and newer studies]. Leipzig, Thieme, 1893, i + 96 pp. (Comprises a Foreword and Nos. 11, 49, 54, 56, 66, 67, 75, and 76 above.)

1894

87. Ehrlich, H. Kossel, and A. Wassermann, Ueber Gewinnung und Verwendung des Diphtherieheilserums [On the production and utilization of diphtheria antitoxic serum]. *Deutsch. med. Wochenschr.* 20:353–354, 1894; *Collected Papers* vol. II, pp. 56–60.

88. Behring, E. and Ehrlich, Zur Diphtherieimmunisierungs- und Heilungsfrage [On the question of immunization and therapy of diphtheria]. *Deutsch. med. Wochenschr.* 20:437–438, 1894.

89. Ehrlich and H. Kossel, Ueber die Anwendung des Diphtherieantitoxins [On the use of diphtheria antitoxins]. *Z. Hyg. Infektkr.* 17:486–488, 1894; *Collected Papers* vol. II, pp. 61–62.

90. Ehrlich and W. Hübener. Ueber die Vererbung der Immunität bei Tetanus [On the transmission of tetanus immunity]. *Z. Hyg. Infektkr.* 18:51–64, 1894; *Collected Papers* vol. II, pp. 63–71.

91. Ehrlich and A. Wassermann. Ueber die Gewinnung der Diphtherie-Antitoxine aus Blutserum und Milch immunisierter Tiere [On the production of diphtheria antitoxin from the blood and milk of immunized animals]. *Z. Hyg. Infektkr.* 18:239–250, 1894; *Collected Papers* vol. II, pp. 72–79.

92. Ueber die Behandlung der Diphtherie mit Heilserum [On the treatment of diphtheria with antitoxic serum]. Versamml. 66 Ges. Deutsch. Naturf. Ärzte (Wien, 1894), p. 187; *Deutsch. med. Wochenschr.* 20:120, 1894 (abstract).

93. Über das neue Diphtherieheilmittel [On the new remedy for diphtheria]. Verh. Deutsch. Ges. öffentl. Gesundhpfl. (Berlin, 26.10.1894). *Hyg. Rundsch.* 4:1140–1145, 1894; *Collected Papers* vol. II, pp. 80–83 (with the title "Über Gewinnung, Werthbestimmung und Verwertung des Diphtherieheilserums" [On the production, measurement, and use of diphtheria antisera]).

94. Ehrlich and A. Einhorn. Ueber das physiologische Wirkung der Verbindungen der Cocainreihe [On the physiological activity of the compounds of the cocain series]. *Ber. Deutsch. Chem. Ges.* 27:1870–1873, 1894; *Collected Papers* vol. I, pp. 567–569.

1896

95. Die staatliche Controle des Diphtherieserums [The governmental control of diphtheria serum]. *Berl. klin. Wochenschr.* 33:441–443, 1896.

1897

96. Zur Kenntnis der Antitoxinwirkung [On the knowledge of the action of antitoxin]. *Fortschr. Med.* 15:41–43, 1897; *Collected Papers* vol. II, pp. 84–85.

97. Die Wertbemessung des Diphtherieheilserums und deren theoretischen Grundlagen [The assay of the activity of diphtheria-curative serum and its theoretical bases]. *Klin. Jahrb.* 6:299–333, 1897/8; *Collected Papers* vol. II, pp. 86–106.

97a. The assay of the activity of diphtheria-curative serum and its theoretical bases (Translation of No. 97); *Collected Papers* vol. II, pp. 107–125.

1898

98. Discussion of "Zur Kenntnis der Antitoxinwirkung" [On the knowledge of the effect of antitoxin] by H. Kossel. Ges. Charité-Aerzte (Berlin, 3.2.1898). *Berl. klin. Wochenschr.* 35:152–153, 1898.

99. Discussion remarks (on Crotin and Tetanolysin). *Berl. klin. Wochenschr.* 35:273, 1898.

100. Discussion of "Ueber das Verhalten des Orthoforms im Organismus" [On the content of orthoform in the organism] by M. Moses. Verh. Ver. Inn. Med. (Berlin, 6.6.1898). *Berl. klin. Wochenschr.* 35:737, 1898.

101. Ueber die Constitution des Diphtheriegifts [On the constitution of diphtheria toxin]. *Deutsch. med. Wochenschr.* 24:597–600, 1898; *Collected Papers* vol. II, pp. 126–133.

102. Discussion of "Inwiefern können allgemeine therapeutische Eingriffe bei Infektionskrankheiten die Heilung befördern?" [How far can general therapeutic intercession promote healing in the infectious diseases?] by A. Wassermann. Verh. Ver. Inn. Med. (Berlin, 4.7.1898). *Berl. klin. Wochenschr.* 35:804–805, 806, 1898; *Ther. Monatsh.* 12:452, 1898.

103. Discussion of "Ueber Leukämie" [On leukemia] by W. Hirschlaff. Verh. Ver. Inn. Med. (Berlin, 11.7.1898). *Berl. klin. Wochenschr.* 35:805, 1898.

104. Ehrlich and A. Lazarus, Die Anämie [The Anemias]. *Nothnagels Spez. Path. Therapeut.* Wicn, Hölder, 1898. I. Abt. Normale und pathologische Histologie des Blutes [Normal and pathological histology of the blood], vi + 142 pp. (2nd ed., 1909). [See also II. Abt. (Lazarus). Klinik der Anämien [Clinic of the anemias]. 1900. ix + 200 pp. and III. Abt. (Lazarus and A. Pinkus). Leukämie, Pseudoleukämie, und Hämoglobinämie [Leukemia, pseudoleukemia, and hemoglobinemia], 1901, bibliography No. 132 below.]

104a. Ehrlich and A. Lazarus, *Histology of the Blood: Normal and Pathological,* Cambridge, University Press, 1900, vi + 142 pp. (2nd ed., 1909) (Translation of No. 104, part I); *Collected Papers* vol. I, pp. 181–268).

105. Discussion of "Ueber embryonale und pathologische rothe Blutkörperchen" [On embryonal and pathological red blood cells] by C.S. Engel. Verh. Ver. Inn. Med. (Berlin, 21.11.1898). *Berl. klin. Wochenschr.* 35:1093–1094, 1898.

106. Ueber die Beziehungen von chemischer Constitution, Vertheilung, und pharmakologischer Wirkung [On the relationship between chemical constitution, distribion, and pharmacological activity]. Verh. Ver. Inn. Med. (Berlin, 12.12.1898); 18:247, 1899. Leyden Festschrift, Berlin, Hirschwald, 1:1–35, 1902; *Münch. med. Wochenschr.* 45:1654–1655, 1898 (abstract only); *Gesammelte Arbeiten* pp. 573–628; *Collected Papers* vol. I, pp. 570–595.

106a. On the relationship between chemical constitution, distribion, and pharmacological activity (Translation of No. 106); *Collected Studies* pp. 404–442; *Collected Papers* vol. I, pp. 596–618.

1899

107. Observations upon the Constitution of Diphtheria Toxin. *Trans. Jenner Inst. Prevent. Med.* 2:1–16, 1899; *Collected Papers* vol. II, pp. 134–142.

108. Discussion of "Die Diazoreaction und ihre klinische Bedeutung" [The diazoreaction and its clinical meaning] by M. Michaelis (*Deutsch. med. Wochenschr.* 25:156–158, 1899). Verh. Ver. Inn. Med. (Berlin, 30.1.1899). loc. cit. 25:46, 1899.

109. Ehrlich and J. Morgenroth, Zur Theorie der Lysinwirkung. [On the theory of the action of lysin]. *Berl. klin. Wochenschr.* 36:6–9, 1899; *Gesammelte Arbeiten* pp. 1–15; *Collected Papers* vol. II, pp. 143–149.

109a. On the theory of the action of lysin (Translation of No. 109); *Collected Studies* pp. 1–10; *Collected Papers* vol. II, pp. 150–155.

110. Ehrlich and J. Morgenroth. Ueber Haemolysine: Zweite Mittheilung [On hemolysins: 2nd communication]. *Berl. klin. Wochenschr.* 36:481–486, 1899; *Gesammelte Arbeiten* pp. 16–34; *Collected Papers* vol. II, pp. 156–164.

110a. On hemolysins: 2nd communication (Translation of No. 110); *Collected Studies* pp. 11–22; *Collected Papers* vol. II, pp. 165–172.

111. Mode d'action et mécanisme de production des antitoxines [Mode of action and mechanism of production of antitoxins]. (Report of Ehrlich's dedicatory talk at opening of the Königliche Preussische Institut für experimentelle Therapie, (Frankfurt am Main, 8.11.1899). *Semaine méd. Paris* 19:411–412, 1899, (extract); *Collected Papers* vol. II, pp. 173–177.

112. Ehrlich and F. Sachs, Ueber Condensationen von aromatischen Nitrosoverbindungen mit Methylenderivaten: erste Mittheilung [On the condensation of aromatic nitroso compounds with methylene derivatives: First communication]. *Ber. deutsch. chem. Ges.* 32:2341–2346, 1899; *Collected Papers* vol. I, pp. 512–516.

1900

113. Ehrlich and F. Sachs. Ueber Condensationen von aromatischen Nitrosoverbindungen mit Methylenderivaten.: zweite Mittheilung [On the condensation of aromatic nitroso compounds with methylene derivatives: 2nd communication]. *Ber. deutsch. chem. Ges.* 33:959, 1900.

114. On Immunity with Special Reference to Cell Life: Croonian Lecture (London, 22.3.1900). *Proc. Roy. Soc. London* 66:424–448, 1900; *Collected Papers* vol. II, pp. 178–195.

115. Cellularbiologische Betrachtungen über Immunität [Cell-biological considerations on immunity]. (Frankfurt, 7.4.1900). *Ber. Senkenberg. Naturforsch. Ges.* 97:147–150, 1900.

116. Ehrlich and J. Morgenroth, Über Hämolysine: Dritte Mittheilung [On hemolysins: 3rd communication]. *Berl. klin. Wochenschr.* 37:453–458, 1900; *Gesammelte Arbeiten* pp. 35–55; *Collected Papers* vol. II, pp. 196–204.

116a. On hemolysins: 3rd communication (Translation of No. 116); *Collected Studies* pp. 23–35; *Collected Papers* vol. II, pp. 205–212.

117. Discussion of "Versuche auf dem Gebiete der Serotherapie" [Experiments in the field of serotherapy] by A. Wassermann. Verh. 18 Deutsch. Kongr. Inn. Med. (Wiesbaden, 1900); 18:566–572, 1900.

118. Ehrlich and J. Morgenroth, Über Hämolysine: Vierte Mittheilung [On hemolysins: 4th Communication]. *Berl. klin. Wochenschr.* 37:681–687, 1900; *Gesammelte Arbeiten* pp. 86–109; *Collected Papers* vol. II, pp. 213–223.

118a. On hemolysins: 4th Communication (Translation of No. 118); *Collected Studies* pp. 56–70; *Collected Papers* vol. III, pp. 224–233.

119. Discussion of "La Leukocytose dans la Variole" [Leukocytosis in small-pox] by J. Courmont and V. Montogard. 13e Congr. Int. Méd., Sect. Path. Gén. (Paris, 1900). 2:184–186, 1900.

120. Discussion of "De l'Origine des Leukocytes dans la Moelle des Os à l'Etat Normale et dans les Infections" [On the origin of leukocytes in the bone marrow in the normal state and in infections] by M.O. Josué. 13e Congr. Int. Méd., Sect. Path. Gén. (Paris, 1900). 2:204–213, 1900.

121. Toxines et antitoxines [Toxins and antitoxins]. 13e Congr. Int. Méd., Sect., Bact. Parasitol. (Paris, 1900). *Wien. med. Pr.,* 33:4–7, 1900; see also Ueber Toxine und Antitoxine [On toxins and antitoxins]. *Therapie der Gegenwart* 3:193–200, 1901).

122. La Leucocytose [Leukocytosis]. 13e Congr. Int. Méd., Sect. Anat. (Paris, 1900). 3:255–266, 1900; *Collected Papers* vol. I, pp. 269–276.

123. Discussion of "Mesure de l'Activité des Sérums" [The measure of the activity of sera] by E. Roux. 10e Congr. Int. Hyg. (Démogr.) (Paris, 1900). *Comptes Rendus Div. Hygiène* 21–27, 1900.

124. Die Diazo- und Azomethin-reactionen [The diazo- and azomethine-reactions]. Lecture "im grossten Centrum der Chemischen Industrie," 1900. (Hitherto unpublished, except for an extended part that constitutes No. 125 below); *Collected Papers* vol. I, pp. 646–650.

1901

125. Ueber die Dimethylamidobenzaldehydreaction [On the reaction of dimethylamidobenzaldehyde]. *Med. Woche.* 151–153, 1901; *Collected Papers* vol. I, pp. 651–653.

126. Ehrlich and J. Morgenroth. Ueber Hämolysine: Fünfte Mittheilung [On hemolysins: 5th Communication]. *Berl. klin. Wochenschr.* 38:251–257, 1901; *Gesammelte Arbeiten* pp. 110–134; *Collected Papers* vol. II, pp. 234–245.

126a. On hemolysins: 5th Communication (Translation of No. 126); *Collected Studies* pp. 71–87; *Collected Papers* vol. II, pp. 246–255.

127. Ehrlich and J. Morgenroth. Ueber Hämolysine: Sechste Mittheilung [On hemolysins: 6th Communication]. *Berl. klin. Wochenschr.* 38:569–574, 598–604, 1901; *Gesammelte Arbeiten* pp. 135–181; *Collected Papers* vol. II, pp. 256–277.

127a. On hemolysins: 6th Communication (Translation of No. 127); *Collected Studies* pp. 88–119; *Collected Papers* vol. II, pp. 278–297.

128. Die Schutzstoffe des Blutes [The protective substances of the blood]. Verh. Ges. deutsch. Naturforsch. Aerzte (Hamburg, 1901). 1:250–275, 1902; *Deutsch. med. Wochenschr.* 27:865–867, 888–891, 912–916, 1901; *Gesammelte Arbeiten* pp. 515–554; *Collected Papers* vol. II, pp. 298–315.

128a. The protective substances of the blood (Translation of No. 128); *Collected Studies* pp. 364–389.

129. Reply to M. Gruber (*Münch. med. Wochenschr.* 48:1669, 1901). Letter to the editor. *Münch. med. Wochenschr.* 48:1808, 1901.

130. Die Seitenkettentheorie und ihre Gegner [The side-chain theory and its opponents]. Verh. Ver. Inn. Med. (Berlin, 16.12.1901). 21:293, 1902 (editor's note); *Münch. med. Wochenschr.* 48:2123–2124, 1901; *Berl. klin. Wochenschr.* 39:18, 1902.

131. Ehrlich and A. Lazarus, Die Anämien [The anemias], *Die Deutsche Klinik,* E. v. Leyden and F. Klemperer, eds., 3:81–97, 1901; Berlin, Urban & Schwarzenberg, 1901.

132. Ueber die Receptorenapparat der rothen Blutkörperchen [On the receptor apparatus of red blood cells], Final Considerations to "Leukämie, Pseudoleukämie, und Hämoglobinämie" by A. Lazarus and F. Pinkus. *Nothnagels Spez. Path. Therapeut.,* Wien, Hölder, 1901, pp. 163–185; *Gesammelte Arbeiten* pp. 555–572; *Collected Papers* vol. II, pp. 316–323.

132a. On the receptor apparatus of red blood cells (Translation of No. 132); *Collected Studies* pp. 390–403.

1902

133. Ehrlich and H. Sachs, über die Vielheit der Complemente des Serums [On the multiplicity of serum complements]. *Berl. klin. Wochenschr.* 39:297–299, 335–338, 1902; *Gesammelte Arbeiten* pp. 282–302; *Collected Papers* vol. II, pp. 324–333.

133a. On the multiplicity of serum complements (Translation of No. 133); *Collected Studies* pp. 195–208.

134. Discussion of "Ueber die Beziehungen zwischen Infektion und der Glykogenreaction der Leukozyten" [On the relationship between infection and the glycogen reaction of leukocytes] by S. Kaminer. Verh. 20. Deutsch. Kongr. Inn. Med. (Wiesbaden, 1902). 20:184–189, 1902; *Berl. klin. Wochenschr.* 39:393, 1902.

135. Ehrlich and H. Sachs, Ueber den Mechanismus der Amboceptorenwirkung [On the mechanism of action of amboceptors]. *Berl. klin. Wochenschr.*

39:492–496, 1902; *Gesammelte Arbeiten* pp. 303–320; *Collected Papers* vol. II, pp. 334–341.

135a. On the mechanism of action of amboceptors (Translation of No. 135); *Collected Studies* pp. 209–221.

136. Ehrlich and H.T. Marshall, über die Complementophilen Gruppen der Ambozeptoren [On the complementophile groups of amboceptors]. *Berl. klin. Wochenschr.* 39:585–587, 1902; *Stud. Rockefeller Inst. Med. Res.* 2:, 1904; *Gesammelte Arbeiten* pp. 326–335; *Collected Papers* vol. II, pp. 342–346.

136a. On the complementophile groups of amboceptors (Translation of No. 136); *Collected Studies* pp. 226–232.

137. Préface to *Le Leukocyte et ses Granulations* [The leukocyte and its granules] by G. Levaditi. Paris, Scientia Sér. Biol., 1902.

138. Neuere Versuche auf dem Gebiet der Serumtherapie [Newer investigations in the field of serotherapy]. *Frankfurter Zeitung* 9.11.1902.

139. Ehrlich and Morgenroth, "Die Seitenkettentheorie der Immunität" [The side-chain theory of immunity]. In R. Emmerich and H. Trillich's *Anleitung zu hygienischen Untersuchungen* [Guide to hygienic investigations], 3rd ed., Müchen, Rieger, 1902, pp. 381–388.

140. Glykogen [Glycogen], in *Encyclopädie der mikroskopische Technik,* P. Ehrlich, R. Krause, M. Mosse, H. Rosin, and C. Weigert, eds. Wien, Urban and Schwarzenberg, 1902/1903, pp. 439–441 (2nd ed., 1910).

1903

141. Comments on "Diphtheriebazillen im Blute und im Behring'schen Heilserum" [Diphtheria bacilli in the blood and in Behring's antitoxic serum] by v. Niessen (*Wien. med. Wochenschr.* 52:2222–2224, 2283–2287, 1902). loc. cit. 53:143–145, 1903. (See reply by v. Niessen, loc. cit. 53:181–185, 1903.)

142. Ueber die Giftkomponenten des Diphtherietoxins [On the toxic components of diphtheria toxin]. *Berl. klin. Wochenschr.* 40:793–797, 825–832, 848–851, 1903; *Gesammelte Arbeiten* pp. 680–726; *Collected Papers* vol. II, pp. 347–367.

142a. On the toxic components of diphtheria toxin (Translation of No. 142); *Collected Studies* pp. 481–513.

143. Quelles sont les meilleures méthodes pour mésurer l'activité des sérums? [What are the best methods to measure the activity of sera?] 13e Int. Congr. Hygiene (Démogr.). (Bruxelles, 1903). *Comptes Rendus, Div. Hygiène* 2: 1903 (8 pp. in German).

144. General discussion of "Mode d'action et origine des substances actives des sérums préventives et des sérums antitoxiques" [Mode of action and origin of the active substances in prophylactic and antitoxic sera]. 13e Int. Congr. Hygiène, Demogr. (Bruxelles, 1903). *Comptes Rendus Div. Hyggiène* 2:12, 1903.

145. Discussion of "Sur la toxine et l'antitoxine diphthériques" [On diphtheria toxin and antitoxin] by Th. Madsen. 13e Int. Congr. Hygiène (Demogr.) (Bruxelles, 1903). *Comptes Rendus Div. Hygiène* 2:32–44, 1903.

146. Toxin und Antitoxin. Entgegnung auf den neuesten Angriff Grubers [Toxin and antitoxin. Response to the latest attack by Gruber] (M. Gruber and C. von Pirquet, *Münch. med. Wochenschr.* 50:1193–1196, 1903). loc. cit., 50:1428–1432, 1465–1469, 1903; *Gesammelte Arbeiten* pp. 727–776; *Collected Papers* vol. II, pp. 368–390.

146a. Toxin and antitoxin. Response to the latest attack by Gruber (Translation of No. 146); *Collected Studies* pp. 514–546.

147. Toxin und Antitoxin. Entgegnung aus Grubers Replik [Toxin and antitoxin. Response to Gruber's reply] (*Münch. med. Wochenschr.* 50:1825–1828, 1903). loc. cit. 50:2295, 1903. (See also Gruber's reply, loc. cit. 50:2297, 1903.) *Collected Papers* vol. II, pp. 391–394.

148. Ehrlich and F. Sachs. Die Darstellung von Triphenylmethanfarbstoffen aus Brommagnesiumdimethylanilin als Vorlesungsversuch [The demonstration of triphenylmethane dyes from bromomagnesiumdimethylaniline as a lecture experiment]. *Ber. deutsch. chem. Ges.* 36:4296–4299, 1903; *Collected Papers* vol. III, pp. 21–23.

149. Betrachtungen über den Mechanismus der Ambozeptorwirkung und seine teleologische Bedeutung [Reflections on the mechanism of action of amboceptor and its teleological meaning]. *In Festschrift zum 60 Geburtstag von Robert Koch,* Jena, Fischer, 1903, pp. 509–526; *Collected Papers* vol. II, pp. 395–405.

150. Ehrlich and J. Morgenroth. Lysine [Lysins]. In R. Pfeiffer, B. Proskauer, and C. Oppenheimer's *Enzyklopädie der Hygiene,* Leipzig, 1903, pp. 58–61.

1904

151. Preliminary comments on "Zur Theorie der Absättigung von Toxin und Antitoxin" [On the theorie of the neutralization of toxin and antitoxin] by S. Arrhenius. (*Berl. klin. Wochenschr.* 41:216–221, 1904). loc. cit. 41:221–223, 1904.

152. Die Bindungsverhältnisse zwischen Toxin und Antitoxin [The binding relationship between toxin and antitoxin]. (University of Chicago, 21.3.1904). *University Record, Chicago* 9:65–76, 1904.

153. The Mutual Relations between Toxin and Antitoxin: 1st Herter Lecture. (Baltimore, 12.4.1904). (Summaries) *Boston Med. Surg. J.* 150:443–445, 1904; *Med. News, N.Y.* 84:760–762, 1904; *Med. Rec., N.Y.* 65:623–624, 1904; *Collected Papers* vol. II, pp. 410–413.

154. Physical Chemistry vs. Biology in the Doctrines of Immunity: 2nd Herter Lecture. (Baltimore, 13.4.1904). (Summaries) *Boston Med. Surg. J.* 150:445–448, 1904; *Med. News, N.Y.* 84:856–857, 1904; *Med. Rec., N.Y.* 65:624–625, 1904; *Collected Papers* vol. II, pp. 414–418.

155. Cytotoxins and Cytotoxic Immunity: 3rd Herter Lecture. (Baltimore, 14.4.1904). (Summaries) *Boston Med. Surg. J.* 150:448–450, 1904; *Med News, N.Y.* 84:906–907, 1904; *Med. Rec., N.Y.* 65:663–664, 1904; *Collected Papers* vol. II, pp. 419–422.

156. Ehrlich and K. Shiga, Farbentherapeutische Versuche bei Trypanosomenerkrankung [Dye-therapeutic experiments in trypanosomiasis]. *Berl. klin. Wochenschr.* 41:329–332, 362–365, 1904; *Collected Papers* vol. III, pp. 24–37.

157. Ehrlich and C.A. Herter, Ueber einige Verwendungen der Naphthochinonsulfosäure [On some uses of naphthoquinone sulfonic acid]. *Hoppe-Seyles Z.* 41:379–392, 1904; *Collected Papers* vol. I, pp. 517–525.

158. Discussion of "Die Serumtherapie vom physikalisch-chemischen Gesichtspunkte" [Serum therapy from the physico-chemical point of view] by S. Arrhenius. Hauptvers. Deutsch. Bunsen-Ges. (Bonn, 1904). *Z. Elektrochem.* 10:661–664; 671–679, 1904.

159. Ueber den jetzigen Stand der Lehre von den eosinophilen Zellen [On the present status of the science of the eosinophile]. Verh. 76 Ges. Deutsch. Naturf. Aerzte (Breslau, 1904). 1:236, 1905 (title only); *Berl. klin. Wochenschr.* 41:1161–1162, 1904 (abstract); *Collected Papers* vol. I, pp. 277–286.

160. Gesammelte Arbeiten zur Immunitätsforschung [Collected works on immunity research]. Berlin, Hirschwald, 1904, xii + 776 pp. Comprises a forword and Nos. 106, 109, 110, 116, 118, 126, 127, 128, 132, 133, 135, 136, 142, 146, above, plus 24 contributions by other authors. (English translations of all papers are in No. 178.)

161. Ehrlich and J. Morgenroth, Wirkung und Entstehung der aktiven Stoffe im Serum nach der Seitenkettentheorie [Activity and origin of the active substances according to the side-chain theory]. *Kolle u. Wassermanns Handb. path. Mikroorg.* Jena, Fischer, 1904, 4:430–451.

162. Foreward to *Die Ehrlich'sche Seitenkettentheorie* [Ehrlich's side-chain theory] by P. Römer, Wien, Hölder, 1904, 2 pp.

163. Ehrlich and H. Sachs, Ueber die Beziehungen zwischen Toxin und Antitoxin und die Wege ihrer Erforschung [On the relationship between toxin and antitoxin and the methods for their study]. *Chem. Novit.* 1:33–37, 65–69, 89–93, 1904/05, Leipzig, G. Fock, 1905 *Collected Papers* vol. II, pp. 423–431.

163a. On the relationship between toxin and antitoxin and the methods of their study (Translation of No. 163); *Collected Studies* pp. 547–560.

1905

164. Letter to Prof. Darmstädter on the need to create a Department of Chemical Research, (Frankfurt, 4.1.1905). Unpublished: copy in the Ehrlich papers, Rockefeller Archives Center, accession No. 87Eh 450, Box 11; *Collected Papers* vol. III, pp. 38–41.

165. Ehrlich and H. Sachs, über den Mechanismus der Antiambozeptorwirkung [On the mode of action of anti-amboceptor]. *Berl. klin. Wochenschr.* 42:556–558, 609–612, 1905; *Collected Papers* vol. II, pp. 432–441.

165a. On the mode of action of anti-amboceptor (Translation of No. 165; *Collected Studies* pp. 561–576.

166. Ehrlich and H. Apolant, Beobachtungen über maligne Mäsetumoren [Observations on malignent tumors in the mouse]. *Berl. klin. Wochenschr.* 42:871–874, 1905; *Collected Papers* vol. II, pp. 472–477.

167. Discussion of "Ueber Trypanosomentherapie" [On therapy for trypanosomiasis] by E. Franke. (Frankfurt, 21.8.1905). *Münch. med. Wochenschr.* 52:2059–2060, 1905.

1906

168. Apolant, H., Ehrlich, and M. Haaland. Experimentelle Beiträge zur Geschwulstlehre: Weitere Erfahrungen über die Sarkomentwicklung bei Mäusecarcinomen [Experimental contributions to the science of tumors: further knowledge of the development of sarcoma in mouse carcinomas] (Apolant and Ehrlich); Experimente an einem Mischtumor [Experiments on a mixed tumor] (Haaland). *Berl. klin. Wochenschr.* 43:37–41, 1906; *Collected Papers* vol. II, pp. 478–485.

169. Ueber einem transplantablen Chondrom der Maus [On a transplantable chondroma in the mouse]. *Arb. Inst. Exper. Ther. Frankfurt* 1:63–73, 1906; *Collected Papers* vol. II, pp. 486–492.

170. Experimentelle Carcinomstudien an Mäusen [Experimental studies on carcinoma in the mouse]. *Arb. Inst. Exper. Ther. Frankfurt* 1:77–102, 1906; *Z. ärzt. Fortbild.* 3:205–213, 1906 (extracts); *Collected Papers* vol. II, pp. 493–511; [See lecture with same title given at the opening of the Kaiserin Friedrich-Haus (Jena, 1908) *Grenzgeb. Med.* 122–148, 1908.]

171. Die Pathogenese des Krebses [The pathogenesis of cancer]. Kaiser Friedrich-Haus (Berlin, 9.3.1906). *Deutsch. med. Wochenschr.* 32:468–469, 1906 (abstract).

172. Bechhold, H. and Ehrlich, Beziehungen zwischen chemischer Konstitution und Desinfektionswirkung: Ein Beitrag zum Studium der "innere Antisepsis" [Relationship between chemical constitution and antiseptic effect: a contribution to the study of "inner antisepsis." *Hoppe-Seyles Z. physiol. Chem.* 47:173–199, 1906; *Collected Papers* vol. III, pp. 64–80.

173. Experimentelle Studien an Mäusetumoren [Experimental studies on mouse tumors]. 1 Internat. Konf. Krebsforschung (Biedelberg, Frankfurt, 1906). *Z. Krebsforsch.* 5:59–81, 1907; *Collected Papers* vol. II, pp. 512–526.

174. Ehrlich and H. Apolant. Zur kenntnis der Sarkomentwicklung bei Carcinomtransplantationen [On the knowledge of sarcoma formation in carcinoma transplants]. *Zbl. allg. Path. path. Anat.* 17:513–515, 1906; *Collected Papers* vol. II, pp. 527–528.

175. Ehrlich and H. Apolant, Reply to "Einige Bemerkungen zur Methodik der experimentellen Krebsforschung" [Some remarks on the method of experimental cancer research] by E.F. Bashford (*Berl. klin. Wochenschr.* 43:477–478, 1906). loc. cit. 43:668–670, 1906.

176. Die Aufgaben der Chemotherapie [The purposes of chemotherapy], Address at the opening of the Georg-Speyer-Haus (Frankfurt, 3.9.1906). *Frankfurter Zeitung* 4.9.1906, 2 pp; *Collected Papers* vol. III, pp. 42–52.

176a. The purposes of chemotherapy (Translation of No. 176); *Collected Papers* vol. III, pp. 53–63.

177. A General Review of Recent Work in Immunity. Included as chapter XLI in No. 178 below, *Collected Studies* pp. 577–586; *Collected Papers* vol. II, pp. 442–447.

178. *Collected Studies in Immunity,* C. Bolduan transl., New York, Wiley; London, Chapman and Hall, 1906, xi + 586 pp. [Comprises translations of *Gesammelte Arbeiten* (No. 160 above); including Nos. 106a, 109a, 110a, 116a, 118a, 126a, 127a, 128a, 132a, 133a, 135a, 136a, 142a, 146a, 163a, 165a, and 177 above, as well as 24 papers by Ehrlich's associates.]

179. Weigerts Verdienste um die histologische Wissenschaft [Weigert's services to histological science], In *Carl Weigert,* by R. Rieder, Berlin, Springer, 1906, pp. 138–141; *Collected Papers* vol. III, pp. 595–597.

1907

180. Chemotherapeutische Trypanosomen-Studien [Chemotherapeutic studies on trypanosomes]. Verh. Berl. med. Ges. (Berlin, 13.2.1907) 38(part 2):35–76, 1908; 38(part 1):56–60, 1908 (discussion); *Berl. klin. Wochenschr.* 44:233–236, 280–283, 310–314, 341–344, 549, 1907; Portuguese transl., *Arch. Hyg. Path. Exotica,* Lisbon, 1:350–389, 1905/1907; *Collected Papers* vol. III, pp. 81–105.

181. Ueber Trypanosomen [On trypanosomes]. *Zbl. Bakt.* 39:537–540, 1907.

182. Ehrlich and A. Bertheim, Zur Chemie des Atoxyls [On the chemistry of atoxyl]. *Pharm. Ztng.* 52:361–362, 1907.

183. Biologische Therapie [Biological therapy]. *Internat. Wochenschr. Wiss., Kunst, u. Technik* 1:No. 4, 1907.

184. Experimental Researches on Specific Therapeutics: 1. On Immunity with Special Reference to the Relations Existing between the Distribution and Actions of Antigens. 1st Harben Lecture (London, 5.6.1907). *J. Roy. Soc. Publ. Hlth.* 15:321–340, 1907; also in No. 203, and in German in No. 204; *Collected Papers* vol. III, pp. 106–117.

185. Experimental Researches on Specific Therapeutics: 2. On the Athreptic Function. 2nd Harben Lecture (London, 7.6.1907). *J. Roy. Inst. Publ. Hlth.* 15:385–403, 1907; also in No. 203, and in German in No. 204; *Collected Papers* vol. III, pp. 118–129.

186. Experimental Researches on Specific Therapeutics: 3. Chemotherapeutic Studies on Trypanosomes. 3rd Harben Lecture (London, 11.6.1907). *J. Roy. Inst. Publ. Hlth.* 15:449–456, 1907; also in No. 203, and in German in No. 204; *Collected Papers* vol. III, pp. 130–134.

187. Festschrift, Das Königliche Institut für Experimentelle Therapie zu Frankfurt a.M. [Festschrift, The Royal Institute for Experimental Therapy at Frankfurt am Main]. 14. Int. Kongr. Hygiene (Demogr.) (Berlin, 1907). Jena, Fischer, 1907, 20 pp.

188. Ehrlich and A. Bertheim, Zur Geschichte der Atoxylformel [On the history of the formula of atoxyl]. *Med. Klin.* 3:1298–1299, 1907.

189. Ehrlich and H. Apolant. Ueber spontane Mischtumoren der Maus [On spontanious mixed tumors of the mouse]. *Berl. klin. Wochenschr.* 44:1399–1401, 1907; *Collected Papers* vol. II, pp. 529–532.

190. Remarks on "Das Wesen der Avidität der … und die Entstehung der Geschwülste…" und "Wachstum … gutartiger und bösartiger Geschwülste" [The nature of the avidity … and the origin of the tumors … and Growth … benign and malignent tumors] by Dr. Orthner. *Wien. klin. Wochenschr.* 20:1329–1330, 1907.

191. Ehrlich and A. Bertheim, Über p-aminophenylarsinsäure [On para-aminophenylarsonic acid]. *Ber. deutsch. chem. Ges.* 40:3292–3297, 1907; *Collected Papers* vol. III, pp. 135–139.

192. Über Antigene und Antikörper [On antigens and antibodies]. *Handb. Tech. Methodik Immunitätsforsch.* 1:1–10, 1907.

1908

193. Das Leberglykogen des Frosches [The liver glycogen of frogs (letter to the editor)]. *Pflügers Arch. ges. Physiol.* 121:236, 1907.

194. Historisches zur Frage der Immunisierung per os [Historical notes on the question of immunization per os]. *Wien. klin. Wochenschr.* 21:652, 1908.

195. Ueber die Genese des Carcinoms [On the genesis of carcinoma]. Verh. 12. Tag. deutsch. path. Ges. (Kiel, 1908). pp. 13–32; *Collected Papers* vol. II, pp. 533–549.

196. Ueber den jetzigen Stand der Karzinomforschung [On the present status of carcinoma research]. Univ. of Amsterdam (Amsterdam, 1908). *Med. Tijdschr. Geneesk.* 1:273–290, 1909; *Zbl. Bakt.* 43:605–606, 1909 (abstract); *Collected Papers* vol. II, pp. 550–562.

197. Über moderne Chemotherapie [On modern chemotherapy]. Verh. 10. Kongr. deutsch. derm. Ges. (Frankfurt, 1908). 10:52–70, 1908; *Münch. med. Wochenschr.* 33:2211, 1908 (abstract); *Collected Papers* vol. III, pp. 140–149.

198. Eugen Albrecht (obit.). *Frankfurter Zeitung* 23.6.1908, magazine p. 3; *Collected Papers* vol. III, pp. 598–600.

199. Ehrlich and A. Bertheim, Zur Diazoreaktion des Atoxyls [On the diazoreaction of atoxyl]. *Chemikerztg.* 32:1059, 1908.

200. Über den jetzigen Stand der Chemotherapie [On the present status of chemotherapy]. Deutsch. chem. Ges. (31.10.1908). *Ber. deutsch. chem. Ges.* 42:1092–1093, 1908; *Collected Papers* vol. III, pp. 150–170.

201. Die Trypanosomen und ihre Bekämpfung [The fight against trypanosomes]. (Frankfurt, 21.11.1908). *Ber. senckenb. Naturf. Ges.* 1:108–111, 1909.

202. Über Partialfunktionen der Zelle: Nobel Lecture [On the partial function of the cell]. (Stockholm, 11.12.1908). Les Prix Nobel, 1909, 19 pp.; *Münch, med. Wochenschr.* 56:217–222, 1909; *Collected Papers* vol. III, pp. 171–182.

202a. On the partial function of the cell (Translation of No. 202); *Collected Papers* vol. III, pp. 183–194.

203. Experimental Researches on Specific Therapeutics: Harben Lecture for 1907 of the Royal Institute of Public Health. London, Lewis, 1908 vi + 95 pp. (comprises a preface and Nos. 184, 185, and 186 above; German transl. in No. 204 below).

1909

204. Beiträge zur experimentellen Pathologie und Chemotherapie [Contributions to experimental pathology and chemotherapy]. Leipzig, Akad. Verlagsges., 1909, vii + 247 pp. (comprises a foreword and Nos. 196, 197, 202, and German transl. of No. 203 above).

205. Über die neuesten Ergebnisse auf dem Gebiet der Trypanosomenforschung [On the newest results in the field of trypanosome research]. Verh. deutsch. tropenmed. Ges. (Berlin, 7.4.1909). *Arch. Schiffs- u. Tropenhyg.* 13 (Beih. 6):91–116, 1909; *Collected Papers* vol. III, pp. 195–212.

206. Zur Einführung [Introduction to the first number of] *Z. Immunitätsf.* 1:1–2, 1909.

207. Die Grundlagen der experimentellen Chemotherapie [The foundations of experimental chemotherapy]. Hauptvers. Ver. Deutsch. Chem. (Frankfurt, 1909). *Z. angew. Chemie* 23:1–7, 1910; *Umschau* 13:839–841, 1909.

208. Ueber serumfeste Trypanosomenstämme: Bemerkungen zu der Arbeit von Levaditi und Muttermilch [On strains of trypanosomes stable in serum: remarks on the work of Levaditi and Muttermilch]. *Z. Immunitätsf.* 3:296–299, 1909;

209. Chemotherapie von Infektionskrankheiten [Chemotherapy of infectious diseases]. *Z. ärtzl. Fortbild.* 6:721–733, 1909; *Collected Papers* vol. III, pp. 213–227.

210. Ehrlich and H. Sachs. Kritiker der Seitenkettentheorie im Lichte ihrer experimentellen und literarischen Forschung; ein Kommentar zu den Arbeiten von Bang und Forssmann [Critics of the side-chain theory in the light of their experimental and literary research; a commentary on the work of Bang and Forssmann]. (*Münch. med. Wochenschr.* 56:1769–1772, 1909); loc. cit. 56:2529–2532, 2586–2589, 1909; *Collected Papers* vol. II, pp. 448–463.

1910

211. Die Chemotherapie, ihre Grundlagen und praktische Bedeutung [Chemotherapy, its foundations and practical meaning]. In *Handbuch der Serumtherapie,* A. Wolff-Eisner, ed., München, Lehmann, 1910, pp. 315–326 (2nd revised ed., 1925, pp. 89–102).

212. Allgemeines über Chemotherapie [General comments on chemotherapy]. Verh. 27. Kongr. inn. Med. (Wiesbaden, 19.4.1910). 27:226–234 (discussion, p. 249); *Collected Papers* vol. III, pp. 235–239.

213. Robert Koch (obit.). *Z. Immunitätsf.* 6:preceding p. 1, 1910; *Collected Papers* vol. III, pp. 609–610.

214. Robert Koch, 1843–1910 (obit.). *Frankfurter Zeitung* 2.6.1910, Magazine p. 1; *Collected Papers* vol. III, pp. 601–608.

215. Ehrlich and A. Bertheim, Reduktionsprodukte der Arsanilsäure und ihrer Derivate. Erste Mittheilung: Ueber p-aminophenyl-arsenoxyd [The reaction products of arsanilic acid and its derivatives. First communication: on p-aminophenyl-arsenoxide]. *Ber. deutsch. chem. Ges.* 43:917–927, 1910; *Collected Papers* vol. III, pp. 228–234.

216. Ehrlich and H. Sachs, Ist die Ehrlichsche Seitenketentheorie mit den tatsächlichen Verhältnissen vereinbar? Bemerkungen zu der 2 Mitteilung von

Bang und Forssmann [Is the Ehrlich side-chain theory compatible with actual relationships? Observations on the second report by Bang and Forssmann]. (*Münch. med. Wochenschr.* 57:851–853, 1910). loc. cit. 57:1287–1291, 1910; *Collected Papers* vol. II, pp. 464–471.

217. 606. Letter to Zelyonoff (*Russk. J. Kozhn. i Ven. Boliezn., Kharkov* 20:92–94, 1910). loc. cit. 20:327–329, 1910.

218. Ehrlich and Hata, S., The preparation for syphilis: a synthetic review. *Am. J. Urol.* 6:503–519, 1910.

219. Discussion on "Ueber die Behandlung der Syphilis mit Dioxydiamido-arsenobenzol" [On the treatment of syphilis with dioxy-diamido-arsenobenzene] by W. Wechselmann. (Verh. Berlin med. Ges. 41 part I:197–198, 1910). (Berlin, 22.6.1911). loc. cit. 41 part II:217–226, 1911.

220. Discussion on "Ueber Syphilis-Therapie" [On the therapy of syphilis] by A. Neisser. Verh. Ges. deutsch. Naturf. Aerzt. (Königsberg, 20.9.1910). 1:172–183, 1911; *Münch. med. Wochenschr.* 52:2158, 1910.

221. Die Behandlung der Syphilis mit dem Ehrlichschen Präparat 606 [The treatment of syphilis with Ehrlich's preparation 606]. Verh. 82. Vers. Ges. Deutsch. Naturf. Aerzt. (Königsberg, 20.9.1910). 2:408–409, 1911, discussion, 409–424; *Deutsch. med. Wochenschr.* 36:1893–1896, 1910; *Klin. Ther. Wochenschr.* 17;1005–1018, 1910; *Korrespbl. schweiz. Aerzte* 40:1051–1057, 1910; *Allg. wien. Med.* 55:457–459, 1910; *Mil. Surg. Washington D.C.* 28:197–205, 1911; *Collected Papers* vol. III, pp. 240–246.

222. Ehrlich and S. Hata. Die Chemotherapie der Spirillosen (Syphilis, Rückfallfieber, Hühnerspirillose, Frambösie) [The chemotherapy of spirilloses (syphilis, relapsing fever, fowl spirillosis, yaws)]: with an introduction by H.J. Nicholls. Berlin, Springer, 1910, viii + 164 pp. (Ehrlich: foreword, pp. iii–v; *Collected Papers* vol. III, pp. 247–248; concluding remarks, pp. 114–161; *Collected Papers* vol. III, pp. 251–281). Translations: St. Petersburg, Ettinger, 1911; London, Hebman, 1911; Paris, Maloine, 1911; Torino, Soc. Typog., 1911

222a. The chemotherapy of spirilloses (syphilis, relapsing fever, fowl spirillosis, yaws). (Translation of Ehrlich's preface in No. 222); *Collected Papers* vol. III, pp. 249–250.

222b. The chemotherapy of spirilloses (syphilis, relapsing fever, fowl spirillosis, yaws). (Translation of Ehrlich's concluding remarks in No. 222); *Collected Papers* vol. III, pp. 282–309.

223. Reply to "Ueber Blasenstörungen nach Anwendung des Präparates 606" [On bladder damage after use of preparation 606] by Dr. Karl Bohac und Dr. Paul Sobotka (*Wien. klin. Wochenschr.* 23:1099–1102, 1910). loc. cit. 23:1131, 1910.

224. Discussion of "Chemotherapie der Syphilis" [Chemotherapy of syphilis] by W. Wechselmann. (*Zbl. Bakt.* 47 (Beih.):129–131). Ber. 4. Tag. Ver. Mikrob. (Berlin, 1910). loc. cit. 223–224.

225. Bietet die intravenöse Injection von "606" besondere Gefahren? [Does the intravenous use of 606 involve special dangers?]. *Münch. med. Wochenschr.* 57:1826, 1910.

226. Remarks on "Die Behandlung der Syphilis mit dem Präparat von Ehrlich-Hata" [The treatment of syphilis with the preparation of Ehlich-Hata] by W. Pick (*Wien. klin. Wochenschr.* 23:1486–1487, 1910). loc. cit. 23:1487–1488, 1910.

227. Au sujet des cas de cécité et des décès imputés au nouveau médicament [On the subject of cases of blindness and of deaths charged to the new medication] (letter to Dr. Netter). *Bull. Acad. Méd.* 64:178–180, 1910.

228. Über die Schlafkrankheit [On sleeping sickness]. *Ber. 4. Internat. Kongr. Fürsorge Geisteskr.* (Berlin, 1910) 4:644–659, 1911; *Collected Papers* vol. III, pp. 310–317. (See "Ehrlich on chemotherapy," *Sleep. Sick. Bureau Bull. London* No. 4, pp. 129–134, 1908–1909.

229. Nervenstörungen und Salvarsanbehandlung [Nerve disorders and salvarsan treatment]. *Berl. klin. Wochenschr.* 47:2346–2347, 1910.

230. Die Salvarsantherapie: Rückblicke und Ausblicke [Salvarsan therapy: Review and prospects]. (Frankfurt, 8.12.1910). *Münch. med. Wochenschr.* 58:1–10, 1911; *Deutsch. med. Wochenschr.* 37:2437–2438, 1911 (abstract); (French transl.) *Clinique, Paris* 6:526, 1911; *Collected Papers* vol. III, pp. 318–336.

1911

231. Pro und Contra Salvarsan [For and against salvarsan]. *Wien. med. Wochenschr.* 61:14–19, 1911; *Collected Papers* vol. III, pp. 337–341.

232. *Grundlagen und Erfolge der Chemotherapie* [Foundations and successes of chemotherapy]. Deutsch. Frauen Roten Kreuz (20.2.1911). Stuttgart, Enke, 1911, 26 pp.; also under title "Aus chemotherapeutischem Gebiet" [From the field of chemotherapy]. *Deutsch. Rev.* 2:149–163, 1911.

233. Permanent action of Ehrlich's new remedy 606 (letter to an American friend). *Mil. Surgeon Washington DC* 28:206–209, 1911; *Collected Papers* vol. III, pp. 342–343.

234. Ueber Chemotherapie [On chemotherapy]. Ber. 5. Tag. Ver. Mikrob. (Dresden, 1911). *Zbl. Bakt.* 50 (Beih.):94–108, 1911; *Fol. Serolog.* 7:697–714, 1911; also prefaced by dedication and tribute to W. Waldeyer dated July 1911, under title "Aus Theorie und Praxis der Chemotherapie" [From theory and practice of chemotherapy]. *Folia serolog., Leipzig* 7:697–714, 1911; Leipzig, Klinckhardt, 1911, 28 pp; *Collected Papers* vol. III, pp. 344–356.

235. Reply to P. Uhlenhuth in discussion on treatment of tumors with arsenical compounds. Ber. 5. Tag. Ver. Mikrob. (Dresden, 1911). *Zbl. Bakt* 50 (Beih.): 124–125, 1911.

236. Richtigstellung zu der Arbeit Fritz Lessers (*Berl. klin. Wochenschr.* 48:1025–1026, 1911) [Correction of the work of Fritz Lesser]. loc. cit. 48:1090, 1911.

237. Ehrlich and A. Bertheim, Reduktionsprodukte der Arsanilsäure und ihrer Derivate. Zweite Mittheilung: über p, p′-diamino-arsenobenzol [Reduction products of arsanilic acid and its derivatives. Second communication: on p,p′-diamino-arsenobenzene]. *Ber. deutsch. chem. Ges.* 44:1260–1269, 1911; *Collected Papers* vol. III, pp. 357–363.

238. Über Salvarsan [On salvarsan]. Verh. 83. Vers. Ges. deutsch. Naturf. Aerzt. (Karlsruhe, 1911) 1:299–315, 1911; *Münch. med. Wochenschr.* 58:2481–2486, 1911; also as "La toxicité du salvarsan," *Bull. gén. thérap. Paris* 162:692–700, 1911; *Collected Papers* vol. III, pp. 364–374.

239. Die Chemotherapie der Spirillosen [The chemotherapy of spirilloses]. *Z. Immunitätsforsch.* 3:1123–1138, 1911 (see P. Uhlenhuth, *Med. Klin.* 7:175–179, 1911); *Collected Papers* vol. III, pp. 375–385.

240. Comments on the previous remarks of Paul Uhlenhuth (*Z. Immunitätsforsch.* 3:1139–1143, 1911). loc. cit., 3:1143–1151, 1911; *Collected Papers* vol. III, pp. 386–391.

241. Concluding remark in the debate with P. Uhlenhuth (*Z. Immunitätsforsch.* 3:1151, 1911). loc. cit. 3:1152, 1911; *Collected Papers* vol. III, p. 392.

242. Preface to *La méthode d'Ehrlich: Traitement de la syphilis* [Ehrlich's method: Treatment of syphilis] by E. Emery. Paris, Doin, 1911.

243. Foreword to *Ueber Neurorezidive nach Salvarsan- und nach Queckzilber-Behandlung* [On the recurrence of neurosyphilis after salvarsan and mercury treatment] by J. Benario. München, Lehmann, 1911.

244. Preface to *"606" in Theory and Practice* by J.E.R. McDonagh. London, Frowde, Hodder and Staughton, 1911.

245. Foreword to *Die Behandlung der Syphilis* [The treatment of syphilis] by W. Wechselmann. Berlin, Coblentz, 1911.

246. *Abhandlungen über Salvarsan* [Essays on salvarsan]. (Compiled and edited by Ehrlich at the request of the *Münch. med. Wochenschr.* München, Lehmann, 1911, viii + 402 pp. By Ehrlich: foreword, pp. vii–viii; concluding remarks, pp. 375–402; also contains papers by other contributors. (Volumes II, III, and IV are listed as Nos. 257, 267, and 274 below.)

1912

247. Über den jetzigen Stand der Salvarsantherapie, mit besonderer Berücksichtigung der Nebenwirkungen und deren Vermeidung [On the current

status of salvarsan therapy, with special consideration of side-effects and their avoidance]. *Z. Chemother.* 1:1–20, 1912; *Ann. Derm. Syph.* 4:186, 1913 (abstract); *Collected Papers* vol. III, pp. 393–404.

248. (Letter to the editor on the danger of using discolored salvarsan solutions.) *Derm. Zbl.* 15:194–195, 1912.

249. Discussion of "Über Verhandlungsversuche mit Salvarsan bei Scharlach" [On therapeutic trials of salvarsan for scarlet fever] by F. Klemperer. Verh. 29. Kongr. inn. Med. (Wiesbaden, 1912), pp. 397–408; 411=412.

250. Discussion of "Über lokale Eosinophilie beim anaphylaktischen Versuche" [On local eosinophilia in anaphylactic experiments] by H. Schlecht. Verh. 29. Kongr. inn. Med. (Wiesbaden, 1912), pp. 414–419.

251. Bericht über die Tätigkeit des Instituts für experimentelle Therapie zu Frankfurt a. M. im Jahre 1910/1911 [Report on the activity of the Institute for Experimental Therapy at Frankfurt am Main for the years 1910/1911]. *Veröff. Med. Verw.* 1:47–61, 1912.

252. Bericht über die Tätigkeit des Instituts für experimentelle Therapie zu Frankfurt a. M. im Jahre 1911/1912 [Report on the activity of the Institute for Experimental Therapy at Frankfurt am Main for the years 1911/1912]. *Veröff. Med. Verw.* 1:62–82, 1912.

253. Ehrlich and A. Bertheim, Ueber das Salzsäure 3,3'-diamino-4, 4'-dioxyarsenobenzol und seine nächsten Verwandten [On the hydrochloride of 3,3'-diamino-4,4'-dioxy-arsenobenzene and its close derivatives]. *Ber. deutsch. chem. Ges.* 45:756–766, 1912; *Collected Papers* vol. III, pp. 405–411.

254. Discussion of "Ueber Wert und Bedeutung der modernen Syphilistherapie für die behandlung von Erkrankungen des Nervensystems" [On the value and meaning of modern syphilis therapy for the treatment of nervous system diseases] by M. Nonne, and "Ueber die sog. Neurorezidive, deren Aetiologie, Vermeidung, und therapeutische Beeinflussung" [On the so-called recurrence of neurosyphilis, its etiology, avoidance, and therapeutic influence] by J. Benario. Verh. 5. Jahresvers. Ges. deutsch. Nervenärzt. (Frankfurt, 1912). *Deutsch. Z. Nervenheilk.* 43:250–270, 270–276, 1912.

255. Über Laboratoriumsversuche und klinische Erprobung von Heilstoffen [On laboratory investigations and clinical trials of therapeutic agents]. Hauptvers. Verh. Deutsch. Chem. (Freiburg, 1912). *Chemikerztg* 36:637–638, 1912; *Collected Papers* vol. III, pp. 412–414.

256. Chemotherapie [Chemotherapy]. Hauptversamml. Kais. Wilh. Ges. Förd. Wiss. (Berlin, 1912). *Soz. Kult. u. Volkswohlf. währ. erst. 25 Regierungsj. Kais. Wilh. II,* Berlin, Stilke, 1913, pp. 345–356; *Collected Papers* vol. III, pp. 443–456.

257. *Abhandlungen über Salvarsan* II [Essays on salvarsan]. (Compiled and edited by Ehrlich. München, Lehmann, 1912, viii + 609 pp. By Ehrlich: foreword, pp. vii–viii; concluding remarks, pp. 568–609; *Collected Papers* vol. III, pp. 415–442; also contains papers by other contributors. (See No. 246 above and Nos. 267, and 274 below.)

1913

258. Moderne Heilprinzipien [Modern principles of therapy]. Senkenb. naturf. Ges. (Frankfurt, 18.1.1913). *Ber. senkenb. naturf. Ges.* pp. 126–129, 1913.

259. Demonstration eines Präparates mit Spirochäten im Gehirn eines Falles von Paralysis progressiva [Demonstration of a preparation with spirochetes in the brain in a case of paresis]. Aertzl. Ver. (Frankfurt, 10.2.1913). *Münch. med. Wochenschr.* 60:443, 1913.

260. Biologische Betrachtungen über das Wesen der Paralysis [Biological considerations on the nature of paralysis]. *Allg. Z. Psychiatr.* 71:830–833, 1913; *Collected Papers* vol. III, pp. 487–489.

261. Ehrlich and L. Benda, Ueber die Einwirkung von Cyankalium auf Pyronin- und Acridinium-Farbstoffe [On the influence of potassium cyanide on pyronin and acridinium dyes]. *Ber. deutsch. chem. Ges.* 46:1931–1951, 1913; *Collected Papers* vol. III, pp. 539–553.

262. Chemotherapie [Chemotherapy]. 17. Int. Congr. Med. (London, 1913). Gen. Sess. vol. pp. 93–111; English transl., London, Frowde, Hodder and Stoughton, 1913, 20 pp. (in German); *Brit. Med. J.* 2:353–359, 1913; *Lancet* 2:445–450, 1913; *Nature* 91:620–626, 1913; *Münch. med. Wochenschr.* 60:1959, 1913 (abstract); *Collected Papers* vol. III, pp. 490–504.

262a. Chemotherapy (English translation of No. 262); *Collected Papers* vol. III, pp. 505–518.

262b. Chimiothérapie (French translation of No. 262); *Ann. Derm. Syph.Paris* 4:561, 1913; *Collected Papers* vol. III, pp. 519–530.

263. Die Behandlung der Syphilis mit Salvarsan und verwandten Stoffen [On the treatment of syphilis with salvarsan and related substances]. 17. Int. Congr. Med. (London, 1913). Sect. XIII, Derm. and Syph. 2:221–231, 1913, discussion pp. 153–154; Sect. II, Nav. and Mil. Med. 2:103–113, 1914, discussion pp. 171–172; *Collected Papers* vol. III, pp. 531–538.

264. Ehrlich and P. Karrer. Über Arseno-stibino- und Arseno-bismuto-Verbindungen [On arseno-antimony- and arseno-bismuth-compounds]. *Ber. deutsch. chem. Ges.* 46:3564–3569, 1913; *Collected Papers* vol. III, pp. 554–558.

265. Erinnerungen aus der Zeit der ätiologischen Tuberkuloseforschung Robert Kochs [Reminiscences of the time of Robert Koch's investigations on the etiology of tuberculosis]. *Deutsch. med. Wochenschr.* 39:2444–2446, 1913.

266. Ehrlich and R. Gonder. Chemotherapie [Chemotherapy]. *Handbuch path. Mikroorg.* W. Kolle and A. v. Wassermann, eds. Jena, Fischer, 2. Aufl. 3:237–271, 1913.

267. *Abhandlungen über Salvarsan* III [Essays on salvarsan]. (Compiled and edited by Ehrlich). München, Lehmann, 1913, viii + 584 pp. By Ehrlich: foreword, pp. vii–viii; concluding remarks, pp. 545–584; *Collected Papers* vol. III, pp. 457–484; also contains papers by other contributors. (See Nos. 246 and 257 above and No. 274 below.)

1914

268. Die Bedeutung der Farbstoffe für die Fortschritte der Medizin [The significance of dyes for progress in medicine]. *Neue Freie Presse,* Wien, 31.2.1914.

269. Deaths after Salvarsan. *Brit. Med. J.* 1:1044–1045, 1914 (letter to the editor; also in No. 274 below, in German); *Collected Papers* vol. III, pp. 485–486.

270. Zum Salvarsanpreis [On the salvarsan prize]. *Deutsch. med. Wochenschr.* 40:1327–1328, 1914.

271. Professor Alfred Bertheim (obit.). *Frankfurter Zeitung* 19.8.1914; *Collected Papers* vol. III, pp. 611–612.

272. Forward to *Gewebekulturen* [Tissue culture] by A. Oppel. Braunschweig, Vieweg, 1914 (2 pp.).

273. Ehrlich and R. Gonder. Experimentelle Chemotherapie [Experimental chemotherapy]. Handb. path. Protozoen, S. v. Prowazek, ed. Leipzig, Barth, 1914, pp. 752–779; *Collected Papers* vol. III, pp. 559–582.

274. *Abhandlungen über Salvarsan* IV [Essays on salvarsan]. (Compiled and edited by Ehrlich. München, Lehmann, 1914, viii + 432 pp. By Ehrlich: foreword, pp. vii–viii; concluding remarks, pp. 417–432; also contains papers by other contributors. (See Nos. 246, 257, and 267 above.)

275. Das Kgl. Institut f. exper. Therapie und das Georg-Speyer-Haus [The Royal Institute for Experimental Therapy and the Georg Speyer House] (On the opening of the University of Frankfurt, 25.10.1914). *Frankfurter Zeitung* 25.10.1914.

276. Bericht über die Tätigkeit des Instituts für experimentelle Therapie zu Frankfurt a. M. im Jahre 1912/1913 [Report on the activity of the Institute for Experimental Therapy at Frankfurt am Main for the years 1912/1913]. *Veröff. Med. Verw.* vol. 4, 1914.

1915

277. Ehrlich and H. Sachs, Impstoffe und Heilsera [Vaccines and antisera]. *Ther. Monatsh.* 29:24–39, 1915.

278. Professor Hugo Apolant (obit.). *Frankfurter Zeitung* 9.3.1915; *Collected Papers* vol. III, pp. 613–615.

279. Introduction to "Ueber secondäre aliphatisch-aromatische Arsinsäuren und deren reduktionsprodukte, speziell 3,3'-diamino-4,4'-dioxy-diphenyl-dimethyl-diarsin" [On secondary aliphatic-aromatic arsonic acids and their reduction products] by A. Bertheim (Bertheim's last, posthumous paper). *Ber. deutsch. chem. Ges.* 48:350, 1915.

280. Ehrlich and H. Bauer, Ueber 3,6-Diamino-seleno-pyronin (3,6-Diamino-xantho-selenium [On 3,6-diamino-seleno-pyronin]. *Ber. deutsch. chem. Ges.* 48:502–507, 1915; *Collected Papers* vol. III, pp. 583–586.

281. Die Antitoxinbehandlung des Tetanus [Antitoxin treatment of tetanus] (letter to the editor). *Münch. med. Wochenschr.* 62:1036, 1915.

282. Ehrlich and P. Karrer, Arseno-Metalverbindungen [Arseno-metal compounds]. *Ber. deutsch. chem. Ges.* 48:1634–1644, 1915; *Collected Papers* vol. III, pp. 587–594.

283. Bericht über die Tätigkeit des Instituts für experimentelle Therapie zu Frankfurt a. M. im Jahre 1914 [Report on the activity of the Institute for Experimental Therapy at Frankfurt am Main for the year 1914]. *Veröff. Med. Verw.* vol. 5, 1915.

1919

284. Die experimentelle Chemotherapie [Experimental chemotherapy]. *Lehrbuch der Mikrobiologie,* E. Friedberger and R. Pfeiffer, eds. Jena, Fischer, 1919, 1:211–226.

NAME INDEX

Subject Index